Julie-Ann Wrightson

Why Can't I Eat This?

Living with
Food Intolerances
WITHOUT Losing
Out on Flavour

For Scott, Zac, Mum, Dad, and Besties,
Without your love and support this book would not exist

First published in 2024 by Julie-Ann Wrightson

© Julie-Ann Wrightson

The moral rights of the author have been asserted.

A catalogue entry for this book is available from the National Library of Australia.

Printed in Australia by Pegasus
Project management and text design by Publish Central
Cover design by Pipeline Design

Disclaimer: The material in this publication is of the nature of general comment only, and does not represent professional advice. It is not intended to provide specific guidance for particular circumstances and it should not be relied on as the basis for any decision to take action or not take action on any matter which it covers. Readers should obtain professional advice where appropriate, before making any such decision. To the maximum extent permitted by law, the author and associated entities and publisher disclaim all responsibility and liability to any person, arising directly or indirectly from any person taking or not taking action based on the information in this publication.

Contents

Appendices

Eating with the enemy

THE EXPRESSION 'YOU ARE WHAT YOU EAT' has been around for decades. It captures the idea that our nutritional choices influence our health and wellbeing, in either a positive or negative way. The food we eat should give our bodies the right nutrients and fuel (protein, vitamins, minerals, fibre and sugars) to function, and if we don't feed our bodies the right materials, our metabolic processes flounder and health declines. Sounds simple, doesn't it? Eat well and you will stay healthy. So why are we seeing a rise in modern lifestyle conditions such as food intolerances, digestive disorders, and hormonal and metabolic dysfunctions? According to experts, we can thank the Western diet and lifestyle.

EATING IN THE WILD, WILD WEST

The Western diet refers to the dietary patterns commonly found in Western countries, such as Australia, the Unites States, Canada, Western Europe and New Zealand. The diet is built on the foundation of refined, ultra-processed foods and beverages, laced with a generous helping of preservatives, artificial colours and flavour enhancers. Hidden refined fats, sugar and salt are thrown into the concoction, creating the every-day convenient foods that we all know and love to eat. Unfortunately, these foods don't really love us. According to the authors of 'Role of "Western diet" in inflammatory autoimmune diseases', these foods containing high fat, protein and cholesterol, and excessive sugar and salt not only 'promote obesity, metabolic syndrome, and cardiovascular disease' – they are also 'possible promoters of autoimmune diseases'.[1]

You will find the Western diet in the takeaway rotisserie chicken you ducked down the road for, the calorie-controlled frozen meal you chucked in the microwave because you were too tired to prepare dinner. It's the Friday night cheeseburger and nuggets you promised the kids, and it's the protein shake and bar you chomped down at work today because you didn't have time to stop for lunch.

Supermarket shelves are overflowing with time-saving, inexpensive, accessible foods such as pre-made sauces, dried fruits, canned vegetables and legumes, frozen meals and pre-packaged dairy. Moisture-infused meats are treated with a combination of mineral salts and water, pumped into the raw meat to produce a tender outcome when cooking, and to prevent bacteria from growing. Cured meats such as bacon, salami, sausages, hot dogs and lunch meats are jam-packed with various artificial preservatives and flavours that are designed to prevent spoilage and intensify taste. These processed foods are widely and cheaply available, making them easily accessible and convenient.

What exactly is processed food – and when did it all go wrong?

Processed food is any food item that has been altered in some way during preparation. Food processing can be as simple as cooking, freezing, pickling or drying a food, or it can be as complex as fermenting, or using pasteurisation or homogenisation processes. Most of the food available today has been altered in some way – even the fresh fruit and vegetables you can buy from the grocer or off the supermarket shelf has been 'processed'. Fruit and vegetables are harvested before they are fully ripened and then sprayed with various chemicals to delay ripening and prevent mould and bacteria from growing.

Food processing has been around for a very long time. As soon as humans began using fire to cook, food processing was introduced as a way to improve the palatability of food and to make it easier to digest. Across the centuries, more complex methods of food processing were developed, such as fermenting, sun-drying, salting, smoking, cheese-making, bread-making, pickling and steaming. The problem is not necessarily in the fresh ingredients used; it's what's been done to them.

The mass scale of food processing and production that we see today is designed to provide a consistent supply of affordable, safe food products to consumers worldwide. People expect appealing textures and bolder flavours in their food, and they expect products to be available year-round, which is why processed food accounts for around 70 per cent of the items you will find in your local supermarket. Many different types of preservatives and additives are added to food to make it look, feel and taste better, and to ensure a longer shelf life.

Most of the time, even processing in itself is not the issue. In most cases, minimally processed foods are not that bad for our health. Minimally processed foods can be stored for a greater amount of time and still remain safe to eat. The enemy here, especially when it comes to food intolerances, digestive disorders and hormonal imbalances, are the ultra-processed foods that are laced with added preservatives, synthetic hormones and flavour enhancers.

Ultra-processed foods are products that have multiple ingredients, including added salt, sugar, oils and fats, various preservatives, flavour enhancers, colours, sweeteners, emulsifiers and any other additive that will allow the food to become more appealing and palatable. Examples of ultra-processed foods include carbonated soft drinks (or soda or fizzy pop), sweetened yoghurts, any sweet or savoury snack, margarines and spreads, breakfast cereals, energy and food replacement bars, energy drinks, candies and cake mixes, instant soup, sauces and noodles, and ready-to-heat products such as chicken nuggets, pies, pizza and frozen meals.[2]

While processed foods offer convenience, taste great, are inexpensive and extend shelf life, quite a number of disadvantages need to be considered. Because processing often removes all natural ingredients and fibre, while adding large amounts of salt, sugar and unhealthy fats to make the finished product tasty and palatable, these foods offer poor nutritional qualities. They are also high in unhealthy additives such as artificial preservatives, colours and flavour enhancers. Many of these are linked to food intolerances and sensitivities, and impact beneficial gut bacteria. They affect behavioural issues and are linked to various health concerns, including obesity, type 2 diabetes and high blood pressure.

Change is coming ... slowly

I know I have painted the modern Western diet as all doom and gloom, and something that's going to eventually make you sick and diseased. That is not entirely the case. In recent years, we have seen a massive shift in attitude towards healthy eating. People have adopted a wider range of eating patterns based on their preferences, tastes, ethical beliefs, health goals and cultural influences. People are becoming more informed about the importance and power of healthy nutrition, and its impact on their overall health and wellbeing. Wellness and self-care trends have gained popularity and emphasised the importance of self-care and nourishing and fuelling the body with wholesome nutritional foods. Nowadays most people are well aware of what constitutes healthy eating. Fresh fruit and vegetables, lean protein, dairy and whole grains are what the experts are telling us to eat to create good health.

Our knowledge of what is healthy food and its availability is not the problem, however. The biggest problem is that we are all time poor, and preparing homemade fresh alternatives most days can seem impossible. It is much easier to duck into the supermarket and grab a box of dried pasta and a bottle of sauce for dinner, than it is to prepare a fresh pasta-based meal from scratch.

The food industry has also started responding to demands from consumers, offering healthier options to meet the growing demand from consumers seeking healthier alternatives. While this is a positive shift towards healthier methods of farming, manufacturing and food processing, when it comes to food intolerances, I believe many problems with processed foods still remain. The complexity of your intolerance will determine what you can and cannot eat.

MY STORY

The reason I'm so passionate about knowing what's in your food is because I know all about the effects of food intolerances – intimately. For years, I was always at the doctors explaining that something wasn't right with my health. I was intent on finding an explanation, and wanted to take back control over my body and regain my optimum health. I was suffering frequent head colds and viruses; my energy levels were very low despite the fact that I was taking supplements. I was bloated, developed hay fever, had a truckload of gut-related problems and was inexplicably gaining weight. I was always feeling rundown, exhausted and just plain blah. My mental health deteriorated, and I was experiencing mood swings, panic attacks and, not surprisingly, felt depressed – suffering what doctors technically call 'general malaise'.

My personal life was in turmoil, so naturally my GP at the time assumed that my chaotic life was the main contributor to my condition, and its array of symptoms. My GP ran a range of blood and medical tests, looking for the possibility of a thyroid issue, or adrenal fatigue, chronic fatigue, low vitamin and mineral levels, and finally any organ function issues. As I said, a range of tests for a range of conditions that might explain the symptoms I was enduring. Every single one of them came back negative. According to these tests, I was perfectly healthy, and my body appeared to be functioning normally. Modern medicine was telling me nothing was medically wrong with me. I was a perfectly healthy 30 year old, so it had to be all in my head, right?

Often people are intolerant to several groups of foods, which makes it difficult for doctors to determine whether their symptoms are caused by a chronic illness or possible food intolerances. My GP was having a hard time finding what was wrong, and because I was not seriously overweight, ill, bleeding, broken or dying, he put it all down to stress and my not-so-happy marriage. In fact, over the next 10 or so years, most of the GPs I visited with the same problems labelled me a hypo-chondriac and were quite patronising. One even patted me on the head and said, 'It's all in your head, Julie-Ann. Go home and relax, there is nothing wrong with you.' I was angry and frustrated. I knew there was something wrong, and I knew it was physical.

So I persisted. Eventually, I found a GP who was as determined as I was to get to the bottom of my problems, and was willing to work hand in hand with my nutritionist and dietitian to find answers. Guided by my dietitian, I completed a detailed food elimination diet (more on that in chapter 1). In total, it took me 12 months to reach a full food intolerance diagnosis. And I won the jackpot! I am not only intolerant to the natural food chemical group (salicylates, amines and glutamates) but also intolerant to wheat, gluten, lactose sulphites/sulphates, propionates, all flavour enhancers (MSG), mineral salts, texturised vegetable protein (TVP), hydrolysed vegetable protein (HVP) and nitrates/nitrates. Phew – that's a total of 13 food intolerances. All processed foods are toxic for me because their ingredients are a chemical cocktail of synthetic and natural preservatives, half of which I cannot pronounce let alone want to eat. That diagnosis was in 2013 – and the years since have been about learning how to live with it!

Since my diagnosis, I have been piecing together answers given to me by various doctors, specialists and professionals (both medical and alternative) as well as my own extensive research while working with NSW Health where I had access to the latest medical research and journals. It's been one hell of a journey, and a constant learning curve that I am excited to share with you.

My journey over these years is why I have written this book. By sharing my experiences and the lessons I've learned along the way, I'm hoping to provide a source of guidance and support for those who are navigating their own digestive challenges and diagnoses. This book is not just about my personal struggles, but also a resource filled with the insights, practical tips and valuable information I wish I'd had when I was first diagnosed. My hope is that you will find comfort knowing you are not alone, and that someone else has faced and overcome similar hurdles.

One important thing I discovered on my journey to recovery is that having a food intolerance diagnosis is not a death sentence for flavour. I am a food lover and I love to cook and eat. When I was told by the allergy unit that diagnosed my food intolerances that I was to have a flavourless life, I became determined to prove them wrong. And I did. Flavour is everything to a food lover and having food intolerances should not condemn you to a flavourless life. So I donned my crooked MasterChef hat and created flavourful recipes from scratch. They are simple, taste great and can be adjusted to suit your own dietary requitements. You can find these recipes in chapter 12.

WHO THIS BOOK IS FOR

This book is for individuals, particularly women, who sense that something is not quite right with their health but have yet to receive a definitive diagnosis. It's also for those who already have a food intolerance diagnosis and are seeking further guidance – because navigating daily life with such a diagnosis can be daunting.

I discovered that the journey to understanding and managing a food intolerance diagnosis often comes with uncertainties. Recognising this is a crucial aspect of self-care and involves making informed choices about what to eat and how to maintain a balanced and enjoyable diet. Adopting a mindful approach when choosing the food you eat is essential. But your choices don't have to be difficult or flavourless; think of your diagnosis as an opportunity to explore new and delicious food varieties that align with your new health goals.

The recipes I have included in this book are not only easy to prepare but can also serve as a foundation for crafting your own meals at home and catering to individual dietary needs. Empowering yourself with the knowledge of flavourful food choices, easy shopping strategies and versatile recipes are all vital steps in enhancing your overall wellbeing and making your journey towards health a more fulfilling and flavourful experience.

HOW TO USE THIS BOOK

The structuring of this book allows you to customise your reading experience – whether you are looking for an overview of food intolerances in part I, practical steps to address and manage your intolerances in part II, or flavourful hands-on guidance in the kitchen in part III. You can navigate the book according to your preferences and needs.

Working out if you have food intolerances – and what might be causing them

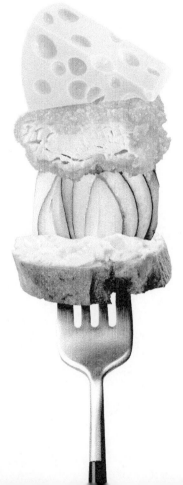

CHAPTER 1

Was it something I ate?

DESCRIPTIONS OF SYMPTOMS FOR FOOD intolerances can be quite tedious and boring to most people, but if you are experiencing them, they are *everything*. Describing to people in detail how distressing my symptoms are can elicit glazed eyes, yawning and people walking backwards to escape me. My colleagues at one time banned all such conversations during lunch time. Hmm.

Symptoms from food intolerances are as individual as the person who is experiencing them. One thing they have in common is that they tend to take longer to appear than symptoms from allergies. The onset of symptoms from food intolerances typically occurs several hours after eating the offending food, but symptoms have been known to appear one to two days later. What I have found in my experience of food intolerances is that this type of sensitivity is responsible for the unnecessary suffering of millions of people and is often misdiagnosed.

Food intolerance is tricky because its symptoms can be identical to other conditions – which commonly leads to misdiagnosis. Physical symptoms include rashes, itchiness and hives, but you could also experience mood swings or anxiety. These symptoms are not always as clear-cut as they might seem on paper, and boy did I find out the hard way.

In this chapter, I provide a quick rundown of some of the common symptoms of food intolerances, before delving into the tricky process of then diagnosing those intolerances.

TRACKING YOUR SYMPTOMS

Some of the questions I am most often asked when I talk to people about my condition are, 'How do you know when you have food intolerance? What are the symptoms?' As mentioned, symptoms can be varied and depend on the individual, but commonalities do emerge.

Some of the more common classic symptoms include the following:

- allergies and frequent infections
- breathing difficulties, wheezing, coughing, asthma
- constipation/diarrhoea
- digestive issues/irritable bowel syndrome/bloating
- headache/migraine
- heart palpitations/general malaise/anxiety/depression
- hormone imbalance/PCOS/infertility
- irregular menstrual periods
- irritability, fatigue, lethargy
- itching, burning and swelling around the mouth and tongue
- mouth ulcers
- nervous tremor
- rash/hives
- runny nose/hayfever-like symptoms
- sleep disturbance/insomnia
- sporadic, persistent itching anywhere on the body
- stiff and sore joints and muscles
- tightness across the face and chest
- unexplained weight gain or loss
- vomiting, nausea, stomach cramps.

Keep in mind that at my 'peak' intolerance periods, I have had every one of these simultaneously. Most people who have a single intolerance will probably get at least a few of these at the same time.

Commonalities in the preceding list imply that food intolerances mostly affect the gut, bowel, digestive and nervous systems. For me, it's like one symptom leads to another, and then the rest follow. Usually I'll start off with the sporadic itching and red blotches or blisters on my face and neck. This is followed by hayfever-like symptoms, including difficulty breathing – plus I have the bonus of what I call 'acid tears', where my eyes water and the tears leave nasty abrasive impressions around my eyes and cheeks. (This is caused by concentrated levels of histamine escaping through my tear ducts. It is very painful, and it takes weeks to heal.) I also tend to puff up like a blowfish, all over. The anxiety follows and involves sporadic heart palpitations; my hands and legs begin to tremble, and I become moody and irritable.

While it took a while to learn not to eat the food that tastes great but triggers a response, you can understand my reluctance to give in to those nasty cravings for the foods that cause these symptoms.

DIAGNOSING YOUR SYMPTOMS

Now that the symptoms are out of the way, let's talk about what you can do about them. I've already highlighted that food intolerances and their symptoms are as individual as the person who is experiencing them, and the bad news is that this also applies to dealing with them. No 'one size fits all' solution is available when it comes to food intolerances; anything is possible (despite what some health professionals may think).

The first step to dealing with the problem, however, is diagnosing it. Health professionals can diagnose food intolerances in many ways, and this is where your personal healthcare preferences come into play. Some people have complete faith in the modern medical and healthcare systems and will visit their GP. Others might avoid a GP like the plague and prefer a more 'natural' approach, and so will see a naturopath or some other 'alternate' specialist, such as a nutritionist, Chinese herbalist or kinesiologist. Or, like I do, you may choose to combine various health practices for a more holistic, whole-body approach.

I don't believe there is a right or wrong way to go about this – your preference, your choice. Obviously, and regardless of their profession, you will want someone who is a professional and whom you can rely on to deal with your symptoms seriously. Initially, I went to my GP because my physical symptoms were quite nasty, and the natural products I was applying to my burning rash and peeling skin didn't help much. In due course, I did end up working with my GP and a naturopath to manage my food intolerances.

Taking the medical approach

Most people start with the medical approach first, and a visit to their GP. Unfortunately, GPs don't have a defined path they can take to diagnose food intolerances. As mentioned, your symptoms can mirror other diseases such as diabetes, anxiety, depression or even an allergy, which makes it difficult to pinpoint the cause.

Hypothetically, let's say you go to your GP because you are feeling bloated and suffering a lot of embarrassing gas, you feel a bit nauseous, your muscles ache with or without exercise, and you are tired all the time. Like any normal modern person, you have of course consulted with Doctor Google. For the symptoms you're experiencing, you've been given a diagnosis ranging from irritable bowel syndrome (IBS) to second stage stomach cancer (which has freaked you out; you think you could be dying).

Likely, you will discuss your diet with your GP, and they might decide to run some tests, just to make sure the issue is not something more sinister. Your tests come back looking good, establishing you are healthy, and your GP concludes that it is possibly diet-related. From here, your GP could take multiple paths; however, the most helpful advice from them would be to refer you to a specialist. Your test results will determine which type. You could see a dietitian, gastroenterologist or a specialised allergy centre – or perhaps, like I did, you will see all three.

Of course, a medical approach involves a lot more than what I have discussed so far. There are too many scenarios I could throw out there to help determine which direction these specialists could take. Ultimately, the decision on where you go next will largely depend on you, your health, your test results and your lifestyle choices. It will also depend on the specialist's area of expertise, their individual professional preferences for treatment and the type of treatment programs available to them.

BABOON SYNDROME?!

Before I move on, I must tell you about one of the most interesting and hilarious medical diagnoses I have ever had. When my food intolerances first emerged, I developed a nasty thigh rash, where my skin was peeling in sheets. My GP believed I had had some sort of allergic reaction and his first choice was to send me to a dermatologist. The dermatologist examined this rash and after taking a sample of my skin, he determined that what I had was an uncommon skin disorder, called ... wait for it ... baboon syndrome! Yes, you read that correctly. Apparently, my rash resembled, and was named after, the distinctive redness of a female baboon's butt! (The medical term for baboon syndrome is symmetrical drug-related intertriginous and flexural exanthema (SDRIFE). Google it. It's real.)

According to the dermatologist, I had had a rare reaction to the various medicated creams I was using to treat my rash. Exotic and fascinating (and painful) though this condition would be to have, this diagnosis turned out to be wildly incorrect, and the nasty burning rash was the start of my food intolerances really rearing their ugly head.

Finding a naturopath or nutritionist

Seeking traditional medical assistance is not the only option when you are trying to determine if you have a food intolerance.

For a more natural approach, some people choose to see an alternate specialist such as a naturopath or nutritionist. Depending on how they practise their specialty, a naturopath or nutritionist will most likely first take a complete case history to find out what your diet and lifestyle is like. They might request some investigative tests, such as a food intolerance blood test or a complete digestive stool analysis (CDSA). A CDSA checks for any deficiencies or issues in your digestive system (looking at good and bad gut bacteria, and parasites).

Once they have assessed the data, your naturopath or nutritionist would then determine if an exclusion diet is necessary, and would start by first eliminating the foods or food groups that showed up in the food intolerance blood test and then slowly reintroducing them as food challenges. This would help them to determine what food or food groups you are intolerant to.

Regardless of who you approach and what their practising methods are, any worthwhile practitioner will suggest some form of supervised elimination diet. An elimination diet is designed to remove certain foods groups or food chemicals from your diet to determine what your body is reacting to. The process could be as simple as eliminating gluten or lactose; if you are reacting to more than just one food group or food chemical, it might be more complex. An elimination diet will help you identify your main dietary issues and, once you know what food group or food chemical is irritating your digestive system, you can heal your body and build a lifestyle plan to suit your dietary needs.

ARRIVING AT THE ALLERGY UNIT

After the exotic, yet amusing (in hindsight), diagnosis by the dermatologist of baboon syndrome, my GP ended up referring me to an allergy unit. We were both unsure as to what was behind my rash, which by now had spread all over my torso and neck and was creeping down my arms. My skin was peeling and burning, I was in distress and the itch was driving me INSANE! I had lived with this for nearly six months. My GP and I, despite all our efforts and testing, were no closer to an answer. I was at my wits' end as to what to do and I was willing at that stage to try anything. I prayed that the allergy unit had the answers I desperately needed.

On the day of my appointment, I spent around three hours with various professionals at the allergy unit. My assessment, by one of their clinical immunologists, included several skin scratch and blood tests. The skin scratch tests would tell them if I had any allergies. Thankfully, the food allergy tests proved negative. I did, however, discover that I had a couple of extra environmental allergies that I hadn't known about. I was glad that the tests so far had not discovered any food allergies. However, further steps were needed in order to rule this out entirely – so I was sent to speak to one of their dietitians to discuss food intolerances and an elimination diet.

STARTING AN ELIMINATION DIET

So, what can you expect from an elimination diet?

The elimination process is designed to help you find out what food you are sensitive to. Just like food intolerances, elimination diets are as individual as the person who is undertaking them. Elimination diets are designed around what symptoms you have, your current dietary practices, and how you can fit the elimination diet into your lifestyle. Some food intolerances are not forever – and some are. You just need to keep remembering that just because you are removing certain foods from your diet for a period of time, that does not necessarily mean it will be forever.

Most people are familiar with removing the more well-known food groups such as gluten or dairy, but you might also need to consider other types of elimination diets.

Here are just a few:

- A **basic elimination diet** is a process of eliminating one, possibly two, food groups or items from your diet. Most people begin with removing gluten, dairy or even eggs from their diet.

- A **FODMAP elimination diet** is the next type of diet your specialist, dietitian or GP will likely recommend. FODMAP is an abbreviation for fermentable oligosaccharides, disaccharides, monosaccharides and polyols, which put simply are a group of short-chain carbohydrates and sugars that are not absorbed properly in the gut. At the time of writing, many experts believe these are the main culprits for most intolerances and aversions.

- A **full elimination diet** is an eating plan that should be designed by a professional – it is not something to undertake unsupervised. This type of diet is designed to remove multiple food groups, food chemicals and preservatives over time, to determine what you are sensitive to.

- A **nightshade elimination** might also be suggested. Nightshades include fruits and vegetables from the solanum and capsicum families. Tomatoes, potatoes, capsicum and chilli are examples of nightshades that are edible fruits and vegetables commonly found in modern diets. Few studies have been conducted to determine if nightshade-edible fruits and vegetables cause health issues. That being said, many professionals out there are of the firm belief that nightshades are responsible for health issues such as inflammation and leaky gut.

It took around five months to complete my elimination diet process. My dietitian and I discussed my symptoms, and what type of food challenges would suit my lifestyle and working week. We decided I would undertake a full elimination diet, and it was hard.

WORKING THROUGH THE ELIMINATION DIET TO FIND MY FOOD INTOLERANCES

I was put on a low chemical diet for two weeks before I could start with my food challenges. This ensured that my body would have time to stop responding to the food that was causing my symptoms. It worked! For the first time in six months, I didn't feel itchy, my skin wasn't sore to touch, and my rash finally disappeared. I cried with relief.

After the first two weeks, I was given a special kit to begin my food chemical challenges. The kit contained 10 individual tablets. Each was either a singular food chemical (one for salicylates, one for nitrates and so on) or a placebo. Neither my dietitian nor I knew which tablets were the placebos and which were the food chemicals; therefore, my own mental reactions or assumptions would not interfere with or influence the results in any way.

These were the rules: I took a tablet while following the low chemical diet, waited a few days and recorded how my body responded. It was a bit like a tango, taking one or two steps forward then one step back. There were days I breezed through with no reaction at all. However, there were other days when my body reacted very badly. I had to wait until my body stopped responding to any residual food chemicals before I could continue and sometimes that could take a week.

I was challenged in ways I could not have imagined, and these challenges were not only physical but also mental and emotional. I discovered just how tightly my feelings were entangled with my food. It wasn't pretty. I had to record every morsel of food that I put in my mouth. There could be no cheating – even though I was tempted to, I simply couldn't afford to cheat because if I did, I would have to start all over again, and that was the last thing I wanted to do. To break the monotony, my dietitian included some food challenges intermittently to the tablet challenges. It was long and tedious and not at all easy. But I survived it. I finished, and I am so glad that I endured the whole process.

Elimination diets are not easy. You can see from my own experiences that when undertaken seriously, they are long, tedious, frustrating and super hard – which is why they are best managed by a professional. Otherwise, on your own, you could be doing more harm to your body than good. In total, it took 12 months for me to reach a full food intolerance diagnosis of the 13 food types I am intolerant to. My next step was to work out the difference between a food allergy and a food intolerance.

CHAPTER 2

Is it an allergy or am I just sensitive?

FOOD INTOLERANCES AND FOOD ALLERGIES are not one and the same. When I go out, ordering food can be quite frustrating after I mention that I have food intolerances and need to request an 'off the menu' meal. Commonly, I am asked what I am allergic to and when I explain that I have food intolerances and not allergies, the inevitable follow-up question is, 'What's the difference?' That's a good question!

Most people recognise lactose and gluten intolerance, but when I mention other types such as salicylates and glutamate, I receive a blank stare. Fair enough. Sometimes it is easier to say I have an allergy than spend 20 minutes explaining what the difference is. However, there is a *big* difference, and it has to do with two of the human body's major highways – the immune system and the enteric nervous system (the digestive system).

UNDERSTANDING ALLERGIES

I'll cover allergies first because I can make this one short and sweet. At one stage of confusion about my symptoms, I wondered whether my physical reactions were due to an allergy. These weird little lumps and bumps that itched, burned and sometimes blistered would appear out of nowhere. My GP and I worked out that when I ate wheat, a few days later I'd develop an irritating, itchy blister, somewhere on my body. It could be anywhere, and it wouldn't stop itching until it popped – a bit like chickenpox. We thought these little irritating blisters could have been a sign of a wheat allergy. (We definitely knew I didn't have chickenpox.) What I now realise is that I am lucky that those little irritating itchy blisters were not an allergy – they were one of the first signs of my impending food intolerances.

An allergic reaction happens when something in your diet or environment triggers a direct response within your immune system. Your immune system thinks it is under attack and goes into defence mode. In response to the 'attack', it produces and releases large amounts of antibodies and inflammation mediators throughout your body. These antibodies are medically referred to as IgE antibodies – and during an allergic reaction they float around your blood stream causing all sorts of havoc, triggering your mast cells to release a 'histamine response'. The problem with having too much histamine hovering in your blood stream is that your body tries to get rid of it as soon as possible. This is why you have a massive reaction like developing hives or blisters or having trouble breathing. It's your immune system trying to release excess histamine the only way it knows how. In severe allergic cases, your body will become hypersensitive and go into anaphylactic shock, which is the last thing you want to happen.[3]

WORKING OUT FOOD INTOLERANCES

Food intolerance, on the other hand, develops when your body starts to react to certain natural or artificial chemicals in food. Food intolerance builds over a period of time. It usually takes two to three days for a reaction to present with a physical symptom, which makes it quite difficult to figure out what type of food is making you sick. Food intolerance does not directly affect your immune system like an allergy does; instead, it affects your enteric nervous system, which causes your nerve endings to twitch and dance and grow additional branches in response to the offending food particles. Your mast cells, which are part of your immunity, release histamine and other pro-inflammatory substances that build up and give you a response as if you have an allergy – but it is not fatal, just really, really uncomfortable.

Food intolerance won't go into 'Terminator mode' and assassinate you like an allergy could. It can scowl at you and say, 'I'll be back' (complete with a cold Austrian accent) – but, essentially, if you accidentally eat something you are intolerant to, you're not going to die! Dramatic? Possibly. But when your tongue is swelling and your airways are constricting, 'I'm gonna die' is the first thing that pops into your head.

The mysterious thing about food intolerances is that so many different types of reactions are possible, and they can impersonate various health concerns. As I mention in the introduction to this book, in the period before I was correctly diagnosed, I was bouncing from doctor to doctor, unable to determine what was happening to my body. I kept repeating that 'something was not quite right' with my health; however, none of them could tell me what. My symptoms were similar to conditions like depression, anxiety and chronic fatigue; my body hurt, my nerves were on edge and I felt run down. All tests came back negative, so I was considered medically healthy. It was assumed that it was 'all in my head'. The GPs I was seeing were good at their job, but at that time I felt like I was being treated in a textbook manner, and my situation did not fit. I like to use the analogy of a square peg in a round hole. I am that square peg and I do not fit into round holes – I tend to break them.

Food intolerance being the trickster of our modern diet, mimicking multiple health concerns, usually results with an inaccurate diagnosis. This was what was happening to me.

The main culprits

While vitamins and minerals are beneficial in maintaining health and wellness, other naturally forming chemicals such as salicylates, amines and glutamates can cause reactions in sensitive people. Indeed, salicylates, amines and glutamates (MSG), along with preservatives, are the main type of chemicals that most people become sensitive to. These chemicals are found in various quantities – naturally in raw and cooked foods, and concentrated in synthetic versions (used for the flavouring and preservation of food). You can also find these chemicals in shampoos, personal care items (such as soaps, moisturiser and skin care) and in some medicines (aspirin, for example, contains salicylates).

Label reading and knowing which chemicals you are reactive to is important because your sensitivity may be exacerbated not only by what you eat but also by the products you choose to wash your hair and clothes with, the type of perfume you wear, your skin care range and even the type of medications you are taking. (See chapter 9 for more on reading labels and knowing what to look out for.)

Thresholds are important

When food intolerance becomes apparent in your body, you will need to determine not only what foods cause problems but also your own personalised balance of reactivity. The allergy unit I attended refers to this reactive response as an individual's 'chemical threshold'. This threshold is basically the degree to which you can tolerate that food or chemical, and it is different for everyone – it depends on how sensitive you are and how much you have eaten.[4] Your threshold also changes over time. If you keep challenging your chemical threshold, continuing to eat foods that contain the chemicals to which you may be sensitive to (salicylate, glutamates, amines and preservatives), your threshold becomes smaller and smaller. You start to become more sensitive, eventually exceeding your 'threshold'. This is like being at the top of a cliff – as you eat these chemicals, you get closer and closer to the edge until you topple into the wide abyss of 'intolerance'.

Here is an example – at breakfast you have a glass of orange juice with no discomfort; however, the strawberry-flavoured yoghurt you had with it (high in salicylates, glutamate and amines) has started to cause a slight reaction. At this point, it's not really a big enough reaction to cause any discomfort. However, for lunch you buy some takeaway food (with a sauce that happens to be loaded with natural and synthetic food chemicals). Your body may start taking notice of the increase in food chemicals and (if you are intolerant) you likely start feeling a little on edge in the afternoon, kind of like you have had a bit too much caffeine and one more cup will tip you over. Your body has reached its chemical load or threshold. When you eat that tomato-based homemade meatballs and pasta you planned for dinner, your body has now exceeded its threshold – and say hello to spasmodic itching followed closely by watery eyes, runny nose, tight chest and an unattractive rash. By now, your nervous system is going nuts and your heart is palpitating, and you're feeling quite emotional and possibly anxious, wondering what the hell is going on. Your body is now twitching and dancing to the food intolerance tango.

Just to emphasise this again for you (and it took me a while to finally 'get' it), symptoms from food intolerances are as individual as the person who is experiencing them. Symptoms occurring as a result of food intolerances tend to take longer to appear than allergies, which will happen instantaneously. The onset of food intolerance symptoms usually appears several hours after eating the 'offending' food, but symptoms have been known to appear one, two or even three days later.

MY SYMPTOMS FROM JUST SOME OF MY FOOD INTOLERANCES

When I have unintentionally eaten foods that contain salicylates, my symptoms don't usually show until the next day. But then I will wake up with a runny nose, tight chest and burning watery eyes; all the usual symptoms for hay fever or the flu. Sometimes I have a cough, but not every time.

If I eat something that has been preserved with sulphites, however, my symptoms are different. My face swells, especially around my eyes, and my tongue feels big and cumbersome in my mouth. My throat and chest tighten, and I find it difficult to breathe. When this happens, I keep reminding myself that it is not an allergy and I'll be okay once I have some antihistamine. I avoid sulphites at all costs because my reactions are so uncomfortable and frightening. As you can see, not knowing exactly what food chemicals were causing my symptoms made it difficult to trace the cause.

My symptoms from eating preservatives are quite painful. My skin becomes red, blotchy and sore to touch, and I can get blisters on my face and neck. I also get the 'acid tears' I described in chapter 1. These reactions are very painful and can take weeks to heal.

At times, my entire body puffs up like a blowfish, and I can have bouts of anxiety and intermittent heart palpitations; my hands and legs begin to tremble, and I can become moody and irritable. My digestive and bowel discomfort is awful, and the degree of suffering usually varies according to the quantity and type of food I have eaten. With physical effects such as these, you can understand my reluctance to give way to any nasty cravings; it took a while to learn not to eat the foods which I loved and tasted great to me. At times, I have given in and said to myself, 'Bugger it – eat it anyway.' After all, I am only human. However, this doesn't happen as often as it used to because the consequences have been punishing.

Continual exposure to food or food groups that are causing a reaction will result in a more aggressive response. Where food intolerances are concerned, reducing your exposure to the chemicals that are causing your reaction will allow your nerve endings to settle and return to their normal level. In some cases, your sensitivities may reduce to the point that they will not return! Unfortunately, this has not been the case in my own situation, but I am continually inspired and compelled to spread the lessons I have learnt.

When I talk to people about my food intolerances, it always amazes me how often others can relate to my story with their own. If it's not themselves suffering, then it's a member of their family, a close friend or colleague. Too many people are suffering, mostly in silence and confusion. For a long time, medical practitioners didn't believe that food intolerances even existed, unless you were obviously lactose intolerant or coeliac. This was because no medical evidence existed to suggest that they were real. It wasn't until the 1960s that sensitivities to natural food chemicals became known and the medical world shifted their focus towards IBS and food sensitivities as a medical condition – and not a psychiatric condition (the 'all in your head' mentality).[5]

Perhaps this greater understanding is because food allergies and sensitivities are on the rise, and more and more people are turning to the health and wellness industry for answers. I was really fortunate to be able to find a balance between conventional medical assistance and alternate practices for my food intolerance diagnosis and management. My GP was open to suggestions from my naturopath and vice versa, which enabled me to have personal input and greater control over my treatment and recovery. This is where my real journey began – when I was empowered to co-design the solutions to my issues, knowing that it was okay not to fit into a textbook case, and that in concert with good medical knowledge and assistance I could lead a 'normal' and very tasty life.

CHAPTER 3

That gut feeling!

GUT HEALTH, THE MICROBIOME AND gut bacteria are today's hot topics. But, back in the '90s when I was experiencing severe bloating, diarrhoea and tremendous amounts of wind (in all directions), it was not the sexy theme it is right now. There was not as wide a range of products on the market to help improve gut bacteria as there is now: kombucha wasn't rocking on every shelf, kefir was not trending and sauerkraut? Sauerkraut was something you ate (if you dared) on occasion with German sausages. Fermented foods for me were pickled onions, gherkins and olives, and my knowledge of gut bacteria and the gut microbiome was virtually zilch. Since it is so integrated into our being at all levels, I now know many researchers even describe the human gut microbiota as an additional organ of our body. At the time, however, I was as oblivious to the amazing powers of the most misunderstood organ in our body as everyone else.

Years later, I have discovered for myself that treating your gut with respect and care can safeguard your whole physical system, reduce the full impact of your food intolerances and, for some people, even prevent adverse reactions entirely. Let me share with you what I've learnt.

GETTING THE BASICS ON GOOD GUT HEALTH

If you're right into gut health like I am, you are probably familiar with the microbiome and the microbes (bacteria) that live there. If you're not too sure, the *microbiome* is the term used to describe the trillions of microorganisms (bacteria, viruses and fungi – that sort of stuff) that live inside and on our bodies, and especially in the gut. While this concept might not be a fun thought if you happen to be germophobic, I like to think of the microbiome as an almost invisible force field for good – a unique ecosystem of living bacteria that protects and enhances my health both inside and out.

When people are talking about gut health and the microbiome, they are generally referring to the human digestive system. Your digestive system starts from your mouth and ends ... well, you know where it ends: your butt. The lining of the intestines is where the majority of your gut bacteria (microbes) live, and the type of bacteria present will either enhance or hinder your health. What you 'feed' your whole system of gut bacteria will determine if you are healthy or if you end up with a nasty overgrowth of bad bacteria, unbalancing your whole system.

Saying hello to your enteric nervous system

Before I take you through the compelling journey of gut bacteria and its mothership, the microbiome, I'd like to take a step back and introduce you to one of the gut's most important internal structures when it comes to food intolerance – the enteric nervous system (ENS). As I mention in the previous chapter, food intolerance has a major impact on the nervous system. It causes nerve endings to expand and grow – if you looked at them under a microscope, they would look as if they were growing additional 'branches' in response to the unwanted food particles. These branches seem to twitch and dance, activating the mast cells, which release histamine, and boom – food intolerance.[6]

As part of the digestive process, one of the jobs of the ENS is to sense the moment food enters the intestines, and then control the coordination of contractional flexes – including the opening and closing of the sphincters (yes, there are more than one). This process helps move digested and undigested food particles through your intestines. Think of it as similar to a production line. When it runs smoothly, and all mechanical parts are oiled and operational, the 'end product' should be well formed. But when there is a malfunction (hello, food intolerance!) it causes all sorts of havoc. Your machinery starts playing up and your entire production line short-circuits (as your ENS twitches and dances). Your goods start backing up (sluggish contractual flexes and sphincters) and toxic gasses become trapped or explode out the rear muffler. The breaking down of food, one of the most important processes in the body, becomes a disaster. And stagnated and undigested food and food particles create the perfect environment for disease, inflammation and toxic bacteria to flourish.

Understanding your gut–brain axis

The ENS assists with the mechanical operation of the digestive process, but this is only one of its important aspects. Another is what is now termed the 'gut–brain axis'. Yep, your gut has a brain and it operates separately to the one in your head. In experiments and studies, experts have proven that if communication is cut off between the 'head brain' and the 'gut brain' (for example, nerve damage cuts off communication), the ENS operates independently. Meaning your body can still go through the digestive process without your brain telling it what to do. Mind blowing, isn't it!

What exactly is the gut–brain axis? In simple terms, the gut–brain axis is the biochemical communication (including signals from gut bacteria, hormones and chemicals) that takes place between the gastro-intestinal tract and the ENS via the vagus nerve. (The vagus nerve is a collection of nerves that connect the parasympathetic nervous system, controlling digestion, heart rate and the immune system, to the brain.)

What this means is that the bacteria in the gut is a governing part of the entire body process. For example, if you are craving something sweet, salty or sour, it could be your bacteria urging you on and not necessarily the neural connections in your brain. When you can't resist that huge piece of chocolate cake, it's not only your willpower that is compromised – it's also your gut bacteria having a hissy fit until you feed them what they want. They make such a fuss that the only way to calm them down is to eat that damn chocolate cake just to shut them up. What's important to note here is that it isn't just your brain telling you what to eat. Cravings aren't just psychological.[7]

Building a healthy microbiome

Gut health is very important when it comes to managing food intolerances. Knowing what works and what doesn't for your body's digestive process is key to managing food intolerances on a daily basis. It's all about being mindful of how your body is responding. Once you understand the digestive process and the importance of the ENS, the last piece of the gut health puzzle are the microbes (gut bacteria) that live there. Our gut bacteria have a symbiotic relationship with our body, and so with our health and wellness, and react very quickly to any changes in our diet, mood or environment.

A 2014 study revealed how diet can markedly affect the human gut microbiome. The study compared a diet of mainly plants (vegetarian or vegan) with a diet of mainly animal-based products, and demonstrated how these different diets dramatically altered the microbiome structure.[8] This simple change in itself 'overwhelms' the bacteria in your gut in a matter of a few days. So, trying out that new keto or vegan diet has significant and rapid consequences. Either one of these diets could potentially enhance your health and wellness (by encouraging good bacteria to thrive) or, on the other hand, cause an overgrowth of bad bacteria (which would leave you feeling pretty terrible and wondering why). Your general health, lifestyle and existing health issues all affect how these types of diets will affect you. This explains why a particular diet may suit one person but have the opposite effect on another.

Essentially good bacteria live harmoniously in the human digestive system. They provide many health benefits – such as assisting the body to properly digest food, synthesise vitamins and minerals, boost immunity, provide energy, promote weight loss and enhance mood and wellbeing. But, it's not all sunshine and rainbows. Bad gut bacteria are what I refer to as rogue microscopic degenerates, and personally I don't want these little suckers growing inside me (and I'm speaking from experience). They are the ones that make you feel awful, influence disease, and cause all sorts of digestive problems and mood disorders (anxiety and depression). Small intestinal bacterial overgrowth (SIBO) and irritable bowel syndrome (IBS) are a couple of conditions that bad bacteria influence.

Food is not the only influence on our gut microbes, with several lifestyle factors also playing an important role in maintaining a healthy microbiome. The gut has a symbiotic relationship with the external environment, and where you live, what you wear, your stress and your mental health are just a few lifestyle factors that influence the health of gut flora. (I cover stress and its affect in the next chapter.)

FROM KOMBUCHA TO MOONSHINE TO FINALLY GETTING IT RIGHT

I was excited when I realised the importance of my microbiome and the influence of gut bacteria on health – and understood how these two elements worked in my body. I had been on a long mission to unravel the mysteries of the microbiome and its relationship to my food intolerances. From everything I was reading, I knew fermented foods and beverages were the most natural and potent way to enhance my gut bacteria. And I knew I was on the cusp of finding out a key element to managing my food intolerances, and a possibly life-changing moment. The biggest problem I faced, however, was that these products were on my never-to-eat-again list.

It was around this time that kombucha (a fermented yeast-based drink) was coming on the market and into the consciousness of people. So, I decided to try it. Now I am the type of person who takes pride in the fact that I can eat and drink just about anything in the search for good health. I had consumed boiled fresh Chinese herbs and barks, ingested naturopathic medicines and drank herbal teas the smell and taste of which could take your breath away, and often looked and tasted like dirt (or worse). But kombucha defeated me. I hated the taste, and I broke out in a rash.

But I was determined! Surely I could tolerate something fermented out there. I was searching for some sort of fermented product that packed the same punch as kombucha and sauerkraut, but without the lengthy fermentation period. I stumbled across another, lesser known product call kefir. Kefir had everything I was looking for: live bacteria and shorter fermenting time, and I was able to make it with filtered water. At the time, kefir water was even harder to come by commercially than kombucha. The only way you could make it was with kefir grains, which four years ago were rare to come by. I attended a gut health summit in Sydney, and this is where I obtained my first batch of kefir grains so I could start the process of making my own.

Kefir water is pretty simple to make. You simply dissolve raw sugar in non-chlorinated water and add the grains, cover the opening with some cheesecloth and leave it in a warm, dark place for around 24 to 48 hours. It is then ready to strain and drink, but if you want to add flavour, you can remove the grains and add fruit, leaving the liquid overnight to ferment a second time. Another thing I love about kefir water was that, after bottling and letting it sit for a week or two, it produces bubbles, which makes it a healthy alternative to sugary soft drinks.

As simple as this sounds, there is still a science to getting it right – and like many things on my self-discovery journey to health and wellness, I got it wrong! I discovered quite by accident that if you leave the fermenting process too long, you end up with a rather potent drink. I was like a bull at a gate wanting to get healthy beneficial microbes into my body as soon as physically possible. I was over it all – all the bloating, burping and wind, I wanted it to go away, and I wanted a cure as soon as possible. In my haste, I (ironically) extended the process. I got the fermenting time mixed up with kombucha and ended up brewing my kefir grains for two weeks instead of the 24 to 48 hours. When I finally did get to try it for the first time, it curled my toes and blew my socks off. Rocket fuel: alcohol in its purest form that tasted like it had been badly cut with methylated spirits. I swear I got a tan from the heat of the body flush that swept from my curled toes to the tip of my nose. I was on fire inside and out! I had unwittingly made my own moonshine without in the least intending it.

It tasted terrible, but this did not deter me. I was determined to get this fermented stuff into my body even if I perished in the process. I needed to be well. I needed my gut bacteria to start working for me by hook or by crook. So, I put up with the burning lava feeling as it coursed its way through my digestive system (along with the molten body flushes) for another month before I realised that I had made a mistake with the recipe. Using my own body as a testing ground has had its ups and downs. (My husband calls me the lab rat – in the nicest way possible.) In reality, I nearly wet myself laughing because it was a typical Julie-Ann moment – determined and wilful.

I am pleased to say that I have perfected the fermenting process now and I was right in the end – kefir water was one of the answers to getting my body back on track to optimum health and wellness without triggering my food intolerances.

Through my ongoing research (and my own trial and error), I now know when I feed my body healthy food, packed with gut-enhancing nutrients, I feel energised and whole – like I could take on the whole world and win. This is the direct opposite of how I felt when I was in the throes of my food intolerance reactions. Research into the connection between managing food intolerances and good gut health and a healthy microbiome is ongoing. For me, it's just something I know – call it a gut feeling!

CHAPTER 4

Stress and histamine and inflammation and hormones – oh my!

IMAGINE YOU ARE SITTING IN peak-hour traffic, late for work, and anxiously watching time tick by. The day before, you found out that your body has been secretly harbouring multiple food intolerances, which means that every aspect of your life is going to drastically change – forever. Panic kicks in and you start to feel quite agitated. Your heart races, your breathing accelerates and your muscles contract, poised, ready for action. Suddenly you yell at the car in front to 'move their arse along' and slam your hand down on the car horn, blasting that pent-up fear and frustration out into the atmosphere. Well, this is what I did the day after I found out I had 13 complex food intolerances. I didn't know how to react. I felt helpless, fearful and angry but, for a fleeting microsecond, that intense, long blast of my car horn and yelling at peak-hour traffic made me feel better.

Stress is a natural physical and emotional response to what life throws at you. Unfortunately, stress – and especially long-term stress – is interwoven with food intolerances. And stress can then combine with histamine, inflammation and hormones to create a pretty nasty cocktail of triggers. When it comes to food intolerances, eating is not the only enemy. Other environmental elements can impact your health in a most unanticipated way, and I cover these in this chapter.

STRESS AND ITS EFFECT ON FOOD INTOLERANCES

We all experience some form of stress from time to time, especially when faced with everyday responsibilities such as family, work and times of uncertainty. Often, stress is related to those awful hair-tearing sessions experienced during bouts of frustration and dissatisfaction. This type of stress is triggered by things happening in life that you have limited to no control over – such as being under pressure from your boss to meet an unrealistic deadline, not having much or any control over the outcome of a particular situation, or discovering (like I did) that you have 13 underlying food intolerances.

Short-term stress can be beneficial to your health and performance. It's that burst of energy that can help you cope with unexpected life events. It helps you to survive (using that fight or flight response) by heightening the senses and improving reaction time and performance. Stress helps to meet those daily challenges and motivates you to reach your goals. But, if the mind and body is in a constant state of stress, it becomes problematic.

You're probably wondering what stress has to do with food intolerance. Quite a bit, actually, since one of the first places stress is felt is in the gut. Stress manifests in the gut in all sorts of different ways – and I'm not just talking about those gut-clenching stomach cramps or nauseous feelings. Internally, stress slows down the digestive process and affects the enteric nervous system (ENS), which is an integral component of the digestive process. As I outline in the previous chapter, the ENS's job is to control the movement of digested and undigested food particles through the intestines. When it is running smoothly and all parts are operating well, nutrients are converted into the fuel the body needs to survive. Like food intolerances, when stress causes the digestive process to malfunction and slow down, stagnant food and food particles become the perfect environment for an overgrowth of nasty bacteria and food intolerance's BFF – inflammation.

LINKING STRESS TO TOLERANCE LEVELS

Personally, I find that when I am under a great deal of stress, my food intolerances 'act up'. This means I reach my tolerance threshold faster, and my body responds accordingly. Food that I can normally tolerate in moderate doses becomes problematic, and I end up with sore and watery eyes, bloated belly, and lots of embarrassing butt explosions.

Stress relates to food intolerance through the release of various pro-inflammatory hormones and chemicals, which include histamine (see the following section). Stress is also linked to gut sensitive disorders such as irritable bowel syndrome (IBS). IBS is a digestive functional disorder that mostly affects the large intestine. It is linked to the overgrowth of unhealthy bacteria, which is why you end up with all sorts of unpleasant gut-related complaints, including enough gas to fill a hot-air balloon. The precise cause of IBS is still unclear, but factors such as long-term stress, food sensitivities, and changes in gut microbes play a major role in its development. Like food intolerance, IBS is linked to the malfunctioning of muscle contractions within the intestines, which causes all sorts of havoc when the body is trying to move food particles through the digestive tract.[9]

THE POWER OF HISTAMINES

I mention in chapter 1 that I have some environmental allergies – these are to mould, pollen and dust. This means that if it is windy and dry (conditions that encourage dust and mould particles to proliferate) my allergies are triggered.

HISTAMINE AND MY FOOD INTOLERANCES

A windy day can cause my histamine levels to rise and, surprisingly, activate my food intolerances. Seasonal hay fever is a nightmare when it comes to my food intolerances. Not a day goes by that I am not responsive in some way, and I find that all through spring, I wish antihistamines came in an intravenous drip. Once elevated levels of histamine are coursing through my veins, my body becomes ultra-responsive, which means I have to watch what I eat and revert back to the basics of my nutrition plan – which sucks big time, because I love food and I hate when it doesn't love me back.

Histamine is a running theme here and is repeated throughout this book. Our bodies tend to have a love–hate relationship with it – well, at least I know mine does. On one hand, histamine is vital because it helps the body to get rid of the things that are bothering it – such as allergens and food sensitivities. Histamine is the first line of defence and starts the process of shoving those pesky pathogens right out of your body.

I feel I can safely say that, if you are reading this book, you are familiar with histamine at some level. You no doubt know that antihistamine medication provides allergy relief from seasonal hay fever, and may have realised it helps with food intolerance symptoms. Histamine seems to be having a really bad wrap here. Yes, it is a big part of the food intolerance tango but, on the flip side, histamine is an essential amine and without it our bodies would struggle to function.

As I've mentioned, stress can cause the digestive system to malfunction, which makes it the perfect environment for stagnant food particles to ferment. Stationary food particles float around your body and irritate your nervous system, which then releases histamine to combat those little suckers. For someone like me who has complex food intolerances, this master plan of misery magnifies food sensitivities and causes all sorts of havoc throughout the body.

ADD IN INFLAMMATION

Another troublesome element to food intolerance's dastardly plan also comes into play here – and that's inflammation.

Inflammation is stress and histamine's feisty big sister – and, man, she is mean. She's fiery, overprotective and quite literally a pain in the derriere. Inflammation leaves a smarting impression and is one of the most uncomfortable symptoms associated with food intolerances. It's the body's attempt to protect itself when it 'misreads' food that it cannot entirely digest. The body believes the undigested food to be a 'foreign invader' (known as an antigen), which triggers the immune system (hello, histamine). The immune system will send out antibodies (protective proteins produced by the immune system) to fight off these invaders. When you have too many antibody-coated antigens floating around in your system for a long period of time, inflammation is the only result.

INFLAMMATION ALERT!

The first sign of my food intolerances is generally an internal inflammatory response. When inflammation hits, I start feeling like I have been in a wrestling ring – and lost. My gut hurts, my body becomes stiff, and I ache in places that aren't supposed to ache. My knees, wrists and ankles throb, and it feels like tiny bolts of electricity are shooting through my muscles. I develop pins and needles in my hands and feet, and I become forgetful and unfocused.

Inflammation is like the pesticide of food intolerance – it seems like a good idea, it's there to protect, but too much becomes destructive and poisonous.

Like histamine, inflammation is often cast in a negative light, but not all inflammation is bad for you, either. In fact, inflammation plays a major role in healing because it fights off foreign invaders (such as bugs and bacteria in infections) and protects and repairs injuries. Inflammation is designed to be short-term, however; when it sticks around and continues to irritate, it becomes a problem.

Long-term or chronic inflammation can become quite serious, and for some people can lead to more serious conditions, such as developing a leaky gut (medically known as increased intestinal permeability). Leaky gut is inflammation's noxious twin sister, and can occur when the digestive process goes wrong. The gut lining is damaged and develops large cracks and holes that allow partially digested food, toxins and bugs to penetrate the tissue around it. IBS, food sensitivities and food allergies have been connected to an increase in intestinal permeability (or leaky gut).

Leaky gut is a controversial topic in today's healthcare industry. Some professionals believe that it is a disease within itself; other researchers suggest that a leaky gut is not isolated, but a condition caused by many gut-related illnesses, including IBS, non-celiac gluten sensitivity and dietary lifestyle choices.[10]

SPRINKLE IN SOME HORMONES

While I am on the subject of inflammation and how it contributes to food intolerances and digestive disorders, I cannot end this chapter without talking to you about female hormones, and in particular menopause and polycystic ovarian syndrome (PCOS).

Menopause is a natural biological process that marks the end of a woman's reproductive years and is caused by hormonal changes, specifically a decrease in the production of estrogen and progesterone by the ovaries. PCOS is a reproductive metabolic disorder that affects the functionality of the ovaries. In other words, it is a disorder that messes up how your ovaries work and causes a hormonal imbalance. The nitty-gritty of PCOS and menopause is quite complex, and I won't go into that level of detail here; however, I can take you through the relationship between menopause, PCOS and food sensitivities.

The hormonal changes that occur during menopause directly affect digestion by producing fewer enzymes and reduced stomach acids. Food travels more slowly through the digestive track, which allows for a longer time frame for the body to fully process what was eaten. This affects the ENS, located in the digestive track. When stagnant food and food particles pass too slowly through the intestines, they create the perfect environment for an overgrowth of nasty gut bacteria, and for chronic inflammation to develop. This is where food intolerances and sensitivities come into play, as the body misreads the food it cannot entirely ingest and starts to think that the food particles floating around inside the digestive track are the enemy. The body sends out its histamine army to protect it, inflammation develops and, for sensitive people like me, food intolerances and digestive sensitivities emerge.

Most people with PCOS will have food intolerances whether they know it or not. Food intolerance is a condition that develops from the hormonal imbalances of PCOS, affecting digestion in the same way as menopause. It slows the digestive process, increases histamine and inflammation develops. However, PCOS introduces one more element to the food intolerance hormonal dance: insulin resistance.

Insulin resistance, where the body's cells have difficulty responding to insulin, is a common feature of PCOS. This can lead to elevated insulin levels in the blood, which contribute to digestive issues such as food intolerances and IBS. Certain types of food intolerances, especially those related to high sugar or refined carbohydrate intake, can lead to unstable blood sugar levels. This can influence insulin production and insulin resistance, which are key factors in metabolic and hormonal regulation.[11]

As the pieces of the food intolerance puzzle fall into place, I believe that not one single element is driving it. Stress, histamine, inflammation and hormones play a major role in the physical development of food intolerance and its symptoms; however, food intolerance is a complex beast and the combination of these factors, along with many different elements, depends on the individual.

PART II

Getting into the nitty-gritty of food intolerances

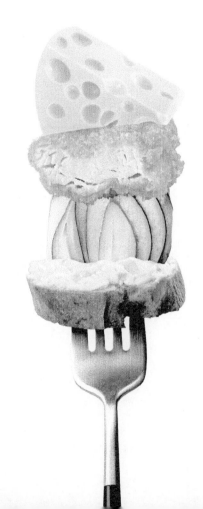

CHAPTER 5

Breaking bad habits: Chemicals

As mentioned in chapter 2, naturally forming chemicals such as salicylates, amines and glutamates can cause reactions in sensitive people. However, these are not the only chemical agents that can cause intolerances in sensitive people. You may find sensitivity can happen when you consume wheat, gluten, dairy, lactose, fructose, artificial sweeteners, nightshades (which are flowering fruit and vegetables from the solanum and capsicum families), food additives and preservatives.

In this chapter, I discuss the naturally forming chemicals salicylates, amines and glutamates to give you a deeper understanding of what each of these chemical agents represent and where they are used in our food. I also quickly run through the nightshades. In the chapters that follow, I provide more insight into other food intolerance triggers, such as FODMAPs, gluten, lactose and preservatives.

SALICYLATES

Salicylates are a group of chemicals that are naturally created in plants and act as an internal pesticide to protect the plant from harmful insects, bacteria, fungus and diseases. They are in a variety of foods, including fruits and vegetables, herbs and spices, nuts, jams, honey, yeast extracts, tea, coffee, juices, beer and wine. Salicylates are known for their pain-killing and anti-inflammatory properties and, as a result, are found in many herbal medications. Naturopaths and herbalists often recommend salicylate-rich foods such as ginger, cloves, turmeric, green tea, and various nuts and seeds for this reason. Aspirin contains salicylates synthetically, in the form of acetylsalicylic acid. They are also found in perfumes, toiletries, cleaning products, washing powders and some botanical oils (such as lavender, eucalyptus and tee tree).[12]

SALICYLATES AND ME

Salicylates are responsible for some of my more annoying symptoms. I know when I have eaten anything that contains salicylates; my eyes water, my nose runs, I itch, and I start to develop other hayfever-like symptoms. I also become restless, on edge and sometimes a bit anxious. This is because the salicylates are affecting my nervous system and inflammation is developing in my body.

It can be quite hard to avoid salicylates – they can be tucked away in popular vegetable powders such as onion and garlic flavouring, and powdered stocks. These powders have very high concentrations of salicylates and may also contain other triggering ingredients (such as wheat, yeast extracts, powdered herbs and anti-caking agents) that are added to keep the powder dry and extend its shelf life. Eating fresh is usually best, but if you are like me and you like flavour, dehydrating your own vegetables and tolerated herbs is a great way of controlling salicylate levels and still keeping your food exciting. I find that if I dehydrate my own fruits and vegetables, including garlic and spring onions, I have more control over the quality of my food and can control how much flavouring I add when cooking.

AMINES

Amines have a close relationship with glutamate. They are a tricky substance because they are in just about everything that is either protein-based or has any intense flavour, such as sharp cheeses, aged beef and red wine (to name a few). Amine intolerance is not something I have. (Thank God! I'd die if I couldn't have a BBQ or eat chocolate anymore.) However, it was still important for me to get to know what they are and how they operate in the body.

Amines (also known as biogenetic amines or dietary amines) are a group of naturally forming chemicals found in food. Amines are usually quickly processed in the body after digestion but, if your body finds them difficult to process due to sluggish or missing enzymes, a build-up can occur, which may trigger an intolerance.

Amines form through the natural breakdown of proteins in our food – that is, with the ripening of fruit and vegetables, in the fermenting process, and when browning, grilling or charring meats and seafood at high temperatures. Amine levels increase in aged foods such as meats, cheese and fish, and are also present in various nuts and seeds, some fats and oils, and fruits as they ripen (including bananas, tomatoes, avocados, pawpaw and olives). You will usually find higher levels of amines in sauces, fruit juices, chocolate, flavoured spreads, nut and seed pastes, jams and fermented products such as beer, wine, yeast extracts, kombucha, kefir, sauerkraut and soy sauce.[13]

Amine intolerance has an adverse effect on the body's neural pathways, affecting not only mood and behaviour but also blood pressure, body temperature and mental functioning (brain fog). It has been associated with migraines, headaches, itchy skin, rashes, heart palpitations, IBS, eczema and depression.[14]

Many different types of amines are produced either naturally or synthetically. People commonly tend to have sensitivity to the following:

- tyramine (found in fruits, vegetables and cheese)
- histamine (found in wine)
- phenylethylamine (found in chocolate).

Tyramine

Tyramine is an amino acid found in both the body and in protein-containing food. Tyramine helps your body to regulate blood pressure and assists with healthy brain function. Foods that are high in tyramine include strong and aged cheeses such as cheddar or blue cheese, cured or smoked meats and fish such as salamis, sausages, peperoni and pickled herrings, and homemade beer.[15]

Histamine

Histamine intolerance is caused by a build-up of histamine levels in the body rather than a chemical reaction to a certain food chemical. In a person who is not intolerant, histamine will break down naturally in their body, nourishing the immune and neurological systems. For someone who is intolerant, elevated histamine levels spreads throughout the body as inflammation and is the cause of some very unpleasant symptoms. Hay fever is a common condition that is caused from elevated histamine levels and presents itself with some uncomfortable symptoms.

Histamine levels in food are hard to measure because these levels depend on how the food is stored, the ripeness or maturity of the food, and cooking and processing practices. Histamine liberators are another element to consider when looking at histamine intolerance. Histamine liberators are foods that are low in histamine themselves but when combined with other foods, help to release histamine into the body. Citrus fruits, peanuts, fish, shellfish and egg whites are known to be histamine liberators.[16]

Phenylethylamine

Phenylethylamine, also known as PEA, is another natural chemical. When ingested, it purely functions as a neurotransmitter by releasing the 'feel good' hormones dopamine and serotonin. Not many food sources contain PEA; however, chocolate, especially dark chocolate, is one such source – which is why when we eat chocolate, we feel good. (It stimulates all those good endorphins in our brains.)[17]

SQUARE PEG AGAIN

Phew, that was all a bit of a mouthful! (No pun intended.)

At the end of my elimination process with the allergy unit, my dietitian was surprised that I was not amine intolerant. She told me that usually when someone is intolerant to glutamate (MSG), they tend also to be intolerant to amines. Amines and glutamate (MSG) work closely together in creating the natural flavours in our food, and it is an obvious assumption that I would have been sensitive to amines. What can I tell you? I am that square peg that is forever being shoved into that round hole.

GLUTAMATE

Glutamate is found naturally in the body and many foods. In its natural state, it is known as glutamic acid and plays an important role in keeping your brain and nervous system healthy. Glutamic acid is produced in the brain and is used as a neurotransmitter (an electrical brain spark), enabling your nervous system to send signals back and forth throughout your body. It is a non-essential amino acid that your body produces without having to ingest it through your food. It plays a vital role in regulating metabolism, memory, brain function, coordination, mood and behaviour.[18] Glutamate is also a natural stimulant and, like all stimulants, when you have too much of it, your body becomes jittery, hyper-alert and anxious, similar to having too much coffee.

Tomatoes, plums, grapes, mushrooms, seaweed, spinach and broccoli all contain natural forming glutamate (alongside salicylates and amines). High traces of glutamate are found in pickles, sauerkraut, some dried fruits and pasta sauces. It is also present in some dairy products, including soft cheeses (brie, camembert, blue), parmesan, flavoured cheeses, yoghurt and flavoured milk.

When glutamate is mentioned, you likely immediately think about the additive monosodium glutamate (MSG), a synthetic chemical added to manufactured and processed foods to make them taste better. MSG is quite toxic for the body. Studies have shown that MSG consumption can cause behavioural issues and contribute to obesity. In Australia, all food sold is regulated by Food Standards Australia New Zealand (FSANZ), which categorises MSG as a controlled food additive. Think of the last savoury flavoured cracker you ate – that intense flavour you tasted is thanks to the flavour additives 621 (MSG) and 635 (ribonucleotides – another chemical similar to MSG). Other ingredients in this type of cracker can also be problematic. Flavour sneaks into manufactured ingredients in many different and hidden ways – another example is powdered foods (garlic, tomato and cheese), which contain naturally formed MSG. I will talk some more on preservatives and powdered foods in chapter 8.

For extensive charts showing levels of salicylates, amines and gluta-mates in various food types, see appendix A.

NIGHTSHADES

Nightshade fruits and vegetables are a diverse range of flowering plants from the solanum and capsicum families. Eating some varieties of nightshade plants can be fatal due to their toxic promoters (for example, belladonna, mandrake root and angel trumpet flowers). Fortunately, these are not edible or used in food, and are more likely to be found in medications.

However, some varieties from the nightshade family are safe to eat and have become a part of our Western diet:

- Tomatoes and tomatillo are considered a nightshade fruit and are a staple part of many diets. Tomatoes are easy to grow and are rich in various vitamins, minerals and dietary fibre. Tomatillos grow in a husk and are like a tomato.
- Potatoes are perennials and a part of the nightshade family. They can be mildly poisonous if eaten before they are ripe, and the skin is still green. (By the way, sweet potatoes are not part of the nightshade family!)
- Capsicums (bell peppers/peppers) are considered the most versatile and tasty of the nightshade fruits, and contain more vitamin C than an orange.

- Hot peppers, such as jalapenos, serrano peppers, and red or green chillies, belong to the nightshade genealogy, and are popular all over the world.

- Eggplant is another member of the nightshade family grown for its edible fruit. Eggplant is this fruit's common name in most countries; however, in the United Kingdom it is known as aubergine and in South Asia and South Africa as brinjal.

- Goji berry (or wolf berry) is a woody bush-like plant native to China and a member of the nightshade family. Goji berries have become quite popular since around 2015 because of their health benefits. Goji berries are a rich source of dietary fibre, vitamins B2 and C and minerals, and are eaten dried like raisins.

Nightshade fruits and vegetables contain a chemical called solanine (a natural plant poison) and some practitioners, mostly holistic, believe that this chemical causes inflammation in those who are intolerant. While no scientific evidence suggests that solanine does or does not cause inflammation, people with arthritis and arthritis-related diseases such as lupus and rheumatism have found that eliminating nightshades from their diets has helped to reduce inflammation and pain.[19]

CHAPTER 6

What the F is FODMAP?

FODMAP IS AN ACRONYM REFERRING to fermentable, oligosaccharides, disaccharides, monosaccharides and polyols. In simple terms, FODMAPs are a group of short-chain carbohydrates (that is, sugars) that aren't absorbed properly in the gut. Removing FODMAPs is usually the first type of elimination diet your specialist, dietitian or GP will recommend when you speak to them about digestive troubles or if you have been diagnosed with irritable bowel syndrome (IBS).

Before getting into why they might do so, let's break this acronym down a little bit further:

- **Fermentable** refers to the process in which your gut bacteria in the large intestine breaks down and ferments undigested carbohydrates and sugars. When your gut bacteria are out of balance, or if you suffer from food intolerances, your body will produce loads of gas. This is the main cause of bloating in your stomach and/or excess wind. The source of this gas is actually the bacteria. Your gut bacteria *love* FODMAPs foods, which are high in soluble fibre (inulin). However, when the gut bacteria eat too much of the fibre (inulin) and their little bellies get too full, they produce gas, which is the main cause of those uncomfortable, and often embarrassing symptoms. (Yes, I am talking about belly rumbles and farts).[20]

- **Oligosaccharides** is a fancy word for fructans and galacto-oligosaccharides (GOS), which are found in various fibrous fruits, vegetables, legumes and pulses. Simply put, they are a group of sugars that the body has difficulty processing within the small intestine. Oligosaccharides assist your small intestine's gut bacteria to flourish. However, if you are sensitive to foods that contain oligosaccharides, you will find they have the opposite effect. Instead, they cause a bacteria overgrowth that results in some very uncomfortable symptoms.[21]

- **Disaccharides** refers to double sugars including lactose, which is found in dairy products and dairy by-products. (Lactose is a combination of glucose and galactose.) If you are intolerant to lactose, you have difficulty breaking down the sugars in lactose due to a missing enzyme known as lactase.[22] (See later in this chapter for more on lactose intolerance.)

- A **monosaccharide** is better known as a single, simple sugar, and this group contains some of the better-known carbohydrates. Glucose, fructose and galactose are all simple sugars and are found in sweet food such as honey or cane sugar. All processed food has some form of simple sugar added to sweeten and balance the flavour.[23]

- **Polyols** are known as sugar alcohols, but unlike the fun alcohol (wine, scotch or vodka) this type of alcohol sugar does not make you drunk (bugger!). Polyols occur naturally in fruit and vegetables, but are also artificially made as low-calorie sweeteners. Sorbitol, mannitol, xylitol, isomalt and lactitol are the polyols that are recommended to be avoided on a FODMAP lifestyle plan.[24]

IBS and digestive issues are becoming quite common, which is not surprising considering what constitutes a modern diet. Experts now argue that uncomfortable symptoms such as gas, bloating, diarrhoea and constipation can be caused by eating FODMAP foods, and this is why your GP or specialist may advise eliminating (or reducing) them from your diet.

As with other food intolerances, these symptoms may not be directly related to what you have just eaten. It can take between 12 to 48 hours for your digestive system to complete its process. For some people, introducing a low-FODMAP diet to your body can bring their digestive system back into balance and rid themselves of all those distasteful symptoms.[25]

For a full list of low-FODMAP foods, see appendix B.

A WORD ON SUGARS

When most people think about the foods that they enjoy eating, sugar, in one of its many forms, is likely a large part of that enjoyment. Who doesn't enjoy a sweet biscuit or two with their cup of coffee, or perhaps a slice of cake or a sweet muffin? (I am celebrating that chocolate is now good for us – chocolate is my go-to sweet fix and I am not too fussed on how I have it.) The delights of sugar have been enjoyed by our ancestors for thousands of years. Kings and queens dined on sweetmeats (such as a date loaf) and candied ginger, sweetened with fruits, dates and wild honey.[26] The ancient Egyptians cultivated dates not only for their dietary and high energy benefits (vitamins, minerals, fibre) but also to use to make sweet wine.

Sugar, in its many natural structures, is a vital ingredient for your body to maintain optimum health. You need sugar in the form of glucose to function. Without it, your brain would not work as well, your muscles would deteriorate, and your major organs would cease to function. Despite all the negative hype around sugar, it is an important element in your diet.[27]

The different types of sugar found in food are as follows:

- Glucose is the body's main source of energy.
- Sucrose, better known as table sugar, is the highly processed white stuff we spoon into coffee and add to muffins, cakes and desserts. It is a combination of glucose and fructose and is made from sugar cane and sugar beets.

- Fructose is the sugar found in fruit.
- Lactose is the main sugar in mammal milk and dairy products.
- Maltose is known as malt sugar and is found in malted drinks and beer.

However, the sugar we know and use today is very different from the sugar or other sweeteners that were used by our ancestors. Sugar, or its evil twin fructose, has been used for many years to help flavour and preserve processed food. The amount of sugar that goes into processed foods is alarming and often hidden behind savoury and sour flavours. Processed foods are cheap and full of artificial ingredients that include fillers, chemical preservatives, colours and bad fats. The combination of sugar and salt is there to improve the food's flavour, so we don't feel like we are eating cardboard.

Our ancestors had the right idea with flavouring their food with natural sweeteners such as honey and dates. We can curb our sugar cravings with sweet fruits, vegetables, nuts and dairy, and now dark chocolate (yay!).

RESETTING MY PALATE

In my own experience, I was quite surprised how sweet nuts tasted once my palette was clean of processed sugar-enriched foods. Almonds, for example, are surprisingly sweet, but most of us are not be able to taste their natural sweetness because of the desensitising effect that excessive sugar has had on our palette. Too much sugar does major damage to our bodies, and it also changes flavour and coats our taste buds. Eating a low-chemical diet changed my palette, and now food I previously thought of as bland has become tastier and more enjoyable.

Sugar intolerance versus sugar malabsorption

Fructose and lactose are among the most common causes of sugar intolerance. Fructose intolerance is a rare hereditary condition – that is, you are born with it rather than develop it. Fructose intolerance indicates your liver enzymes operate deficiently and are unable to successfully break down this type of sugar. Having a fructose intolerance can lead to serious medical issues such as liver and kidney failure, and needs to be properly diagnosed by a medical professional.

Lactose intolerance is one of the better-known sugar intolerances and is a result of the individual's inability to properly digest lactose, which is the sugar found in the milk of mammals and other dairy-like products. (See the following section for more on lactose intolerance.)

Sugar malabsorption, on the other hand, is the body's inability to break down sugars in the small intestine. Sugar malabsorption occurs at the point where the sugar moves through your small intestine into your larger intestine. Your gut bacteria use the undigested sugar as food, and in that process produce gasses. The result is painful bloating, diarrhoea and flatulence.[28]

Lactose intolerance

Gas, bloating, nausea and vomiting are common symptoms of lactose intolerance. These are caused by the body's inability to break down the naturally occurring sugar lactose, found in most dairy products, due to it not producing enough of the gut enzyme lactase. A study conducted in Australia between 2011 and 2015 by Roy Morgan Research found that a quarter of a million Australians report being lactose intolerant. Women across all ages appear to be more receptive to it than men, with the condition affecting 6.2 per cent of women aged over 18. Worldwide, around 65 per cent of people have a reduced ability to digest lactose after infancy. (It is common in people of East Asian, West African, Arab, Jewish, Greek and Italian descent, due to their more habitual use of fermented milk products as an important food source.)[29]

Lactose is not just found in dairy products. Millions of tonnes of dairy by-products, including whey, protein isolate (used in body building and weight loss protein powders), skim milk powder and milk solids, are added as cheap ingredients to processed foods.[30]

ADDING LACTOSE INTOLERANCE TO THE MIX

All my life, I have loved and eaten dairy in many of its delicious forms – including hard cheese (not the smelly kind), soft cheese, milk, yoghurt and ice cream. I ate and loved it all. Not long after I completed my food challenges through the Allergy Unit, lactose intolerance raised its ugly head. I was shattered. As far as I was concerned, dairy had not been an issue and this particular intolerance did not come out during my elimination process, or so I thought. A few months after the end of my supervised diet, however, I began to react to dairy. At times, I would vomit after I had milk or yoghurt. I mentioned this to my specialist and he, in turn, diagnosed me with lactose intolerance (joy!). So, as it turns out, the elimination diet itself triggered my lactose intolerance. It is my belief that my system was becoming highly sensitised and that the elimination diet heightened this sensitivity – and lactose was in the firing line!

I discovered after my diagnosis that lactose is also present in commercially produced soups, salad dressings and sauces (powdered and liquid), and is often used as a substance filler in around 20 per cent of medications. More recently, I identified that a medication I have been taking for the last five years contains lactose, which has caused me endless suffering. Before realising this, I had been having difficulty in identifying the cause of my constant stomach bloat and pain. My discovery explained a lot.

Some people can tolerate small amounts of lactose and can eat in the low-tolerance range – for example, hard and aged cheeses generally have lower levels of lactose. Yoghurts are said to be digestible because the bacteria strains eat the lactose, which can help our bodies break it down more efficiently. I tried that and it wasn't pretty, but that's not to say that it won't work for other people.

Whether you can eat some diary or need to choose lactose-free products, you may still need to check the levels of salicylates, amines and glutamates in the products you're considering. See appendix A for a table outlining the levels of these chemicals in dairy, lactose-free and dairy alternative foods.

ARE INTENSE (ARTIFICIAL) SWEETENERS BETTER FOR YOU?

The sugar-free revolution is upon us! People are now interested in leading a healthier lifestyle, and reducing their sugar intake is often top on their list. The current knowledge we have on lifestyle diseases (including type 2 diabetes and obesity) and how to prevent them has grown and it appears to be influencing most people to adopt a low-sugar lifestyle. In their quest, many people have shifted from consuming sugar to using an alternative sweetener. On top of this, a wider array of foods and beverages contain some form of artificial sweetener. You can find them in a variety of commercially available baked goods (cakes, muffins and health bars, to name a few), yoghurts, dairy desserts, jelly crystals, confectionary, chewing gum – basically, anything that has been labelled 'sugar free' or 'low calorie' has some form of artificial sweetener.

Intense sweeteners are around 20,000 times sweeter than table sugar and for decades have been under scrutiny, with studies suggesting that they are not as good for us as they seem. Recent studies have shown that intense sweeteners are linked to the growing pandemic of obesity and type 2 diabetes. Eran Elinav, a researcher at the Weizmann Institute of Science in Rehovot, Israel, says, 'The most shocking result is that the use of sweeteners aimed at preventing diabetes might actually be contributing to and possibly driving the epidemic that it aims to prevent.'[31]

These studies suggested that intense sweeteners change how your body processes fat within your metabolism and end up producing the same type of health consequences as sugar. Intense sweeteners trick the body into believing it has had something sweet to eat; however, when our body realises it has been fooled, it tries to find the energy source elsewhere (like your muscles). Researchers have found evidence of protein breakdown within the blood of the test subjects – which basically means that the test subjects were burning muscle tissue as opposed to body fat as a source of energy.[32]

Intense sweeteners have also been linked to the misdiagnosis of IBS due to their laxative effect. Current Australian food regulations require that artificial sweeteners used in our food must be labelled with appropriate warnings, such as 'excessive consumption may have a laxative effect'. It is not uncommon to miss this message, however, unless you are an avid label reader.

The connection between intense sweeteners and 'stomach upsets' is something that most people don't think about. Why would you think that a stick of sugar-free chewing gum and a sugar-free protein bar would be the cause of your stomach bloat or excessive cramping? Most of us wouldn't, because we don't link the sugar-free food as being 'excessive'.

Artificial sweeteners are often combined, so don't be fooled into thinking that you are only consuming one sweetening agent. No-sugar soft drinks (or sodas) are examples of this. These drinks often contain a combination of acesulphame K (950) and aspartame (951). The code numbering of these additives is indicated on the ingredients list; however, the quantities are not. Unless you know what the sweeteners 950 and 951 are, you are not going to know that you are drinking aspartame, nor do you know how much you are having per can. (Australian labels do not have to indicate how much sweetener is used per ml.) Without this vital piece of information, you cannot make an informed decision around how much 'sugar-free' or 'diet' items you're consuming per day.

The sugar alternatives approved by Food Standards Australia New Zealand (FSANZ) for use in our food today are divided into three categories:

1. artificial sweeteners
2. nutritive sweeteners
3. natural intense sweeteners.

Artificial sweeteners

Artificial sweeteners are used as a sugar alternative and have a calorie or kilojoule rating of zero. Zero-calorie food and beverages are obviously extremely popular with the diet and weight loss industries, and these sweeteners are a key ingredient in many 'diet' labelled products. Artificial sweeteners are used in diet soft drinks, jellies, yoghurts, ice creams, chewing gum, confectionary and desserts, and commonly labelled as 'diet', low joule', 'no sugar' or 'sugar free' products. Interestingly, only a handful of artificial sweeteners are approved by FSANZ – see appendix C.

Nutritive sweeteners

Nutritive sweeteners are used as flavour enhancers. They have some calories, but far fewer than sugar and do provide energy to our bodies through carbohydrates (like fructose – fruit sugars). Nutritive sweeteners are used to sweeten our food and drinks and can be used as a table-top sweetener (Xylitol, for example, can be used as a table-top sugar). As with artificial sweeteners, they are used to flavour and sweeten diet soft drinks, jellies, yoghurts, ice creams, chewing gum, confectionary and deserts.

Natural intense sweeteners

Natural intense sweeteners have recently been recognised as an approved flavour enhancing substance. The most common goes by the name of stevia (960). Stevia is extracted from the *Stevia rebaudiana* plant, which is a shrub from the chrysanthemum family and native to South America. Stevia is around 200 to 300 times sweeter than regular sugar and has no calorie content. It is becoming more popular as a sweetening agent and is mostly used in soft drinks and flavoured waters. Stevia can also be used in baked goods, dairy products and confectionary, as a table-top sugar and is available in liquid form.

Stevia accounts for around 30 per cent of the low-kilojoule sweetener market in Australia and New Zealand and is advertised as a 'natural sweetener'. However, the question about the 'natural' properties of stevia continues to be debated. Dr Alan Barclay, formerly of Diabetics Australia and spokesman for the Dietitians Association of Australia, says that stevia may not be quite as 'natural' as the marketing would have us believe. We do not eat stevia in its natural form. According to Barclay, stevia powder 'is a highly refined extract, blended with sugar alcohol and bulked up with maltodextrin … To get it table-top sweet, it's bulked out with other carbohydrates, which are calorific.' (Maltodextrin is a white powder made from corn, rice and potato starch.)[33]

For a full list of the artificial and nutritive sweeteners approved for consumption by FSANZ, see appendix C. The tables provided are a good reference, but you do not have to memorise every artificial sweetener on the market or their identity numbers to make an informed decision. The way I remember is if the label says 'no sugar', 'low calorie' or anything diet, chances are one or more of these nasty ingredients will be in it. When I must choose between having food sweetened with sugar, and food sweetened artificially, I pick sugar every time (while still being observant of the amount of sugar per serving).

CHAPTER 7

What's with non-coeliac gluten sensitivity?

Wheat and wheat by-products are in almost *everything*! And I am not just talking about food here; I'm also talking about skincare, make-up, dental products, soaps and body washes, shampoos, conditioners, medications, vitamins and mineral supplements, protein and weight management shakes, and some sunscreens. I kid you not!

In this chapter, I run through why this might be a problem for people with coeliac disease and gluten sensitivity, and what scientists believe could be behind these issues.

WHY GLUTEN CAN BE A PROBLEM

The deluge of wheat has become a problem for people like me who are sensitive to gluten – a protein found in wheat, barley, rye and oats. Gluten-containing grains are a major part of the modern Western diet, with wheat and wheat by-products (fillers, starches and thickeners) the shining stars. Over recent years, experts have been seeing a rise in gluten-related autoimmune conditions such as coeliac disease, psoriasis and rheumatoid arthritis. Now there is a new kid on the block: non-coeliac gluten sensitivity (NCGS).

NCGS is the fancy medical term for gluten intolerance, and it occurs when your body finds it difficult to break down gluten, similar to coeliac disease. Gluten sensitivity affects around 10 per cent of the world's population – although experts believe that most of that percentage is due to lifestyle choices (that is, people choosing to omit gluten from their diet even when they do not suffer an intolerance). In the low-carb world, modern diets target grain-free eating, and wheat-based products are on their kill list. Many people have been switching to gluten-free diets to lose weight, reduce inflammation and boost energy, which are all fantastic reasons to improve your overall health. However, experts believe that, for most people, eliminating grains may not be the best dietary choice. They are concerned that people who are not sensitive to gluten or do not have coeliac disease are not receiving the nutritional and caloric benefits their body needs.[34]

Coeliac disease occurs when the immune system thinks that gluten is the enemy and goes into defence mode. Your immune system attacks the protein when it reaches the small intestine, causing damage to the lining and finger-like projections known as villi. (Your body absorbs the nutrients from food via these villi.) The villi become inflamed and flattened, causing all sorts of health problems. People with coeliac disease have serious issues with vitamin and mineral deficiencies, experience sudden weight loss or weight gain, have bone and joint pain, suffer from fatigue and a foggy brain, and have digestive complications including cramping, bloating and abdominal pain. In children, there is a failure to thrive and delays with puberty. As you can see, coeliac disease is quite serious and can have devastating effects on the body.

MY JOURNEY TO GLUTEN FREE

It has taken me 25 years to become completely gluten free. I experienced a slew of awful and uncomfortable symptoms after the birth of my son in

1997. At that time, I could not definitively associate these symptoms with anything specific I was or was not eating, and I had no idea that my love of bread and bread-type products could be the cause of so much pain and discomfort. My GP at the time was very thorough in his investigations; I became a complex puzzle that he was determined to solve. Eventually he looked at my nutrition, even though I had mentioned to him that I was following a well-known diet regime to try to deal with my unexplained weight gain. On his advice, I recorded my food intake for a few weeks, and we discovered that I was eating a lot of wheat in one form or another. Even though I was following a controlled and planned diet, many of my food choices included products that contained wheat and gluten – such as rolled oats, yoghurts with thickeners, rice biscuits, low-fat muffins and natural wraps.

Eliminating gluten was a long shot, but I gave it a go and I am so glad that I did. I found it exceedingly difficult to give up my beloved bread and, back then, few gluten free options were available that tasted even remotely nice. Most were like munching on flavourless cardboard. However, I gave it a go, and found that after a month or two I did feel better. My GP at the time and I worked out that I could tolerate gluten in smaller doses, which meant that if I had a bread roll for lunch one day, I would be fine, but could not eat gluten again for the next few days. As the years and decades grew, so did my intolerance and now I am completely gluten free. I find that if I have even the smallest amount of gluten (say, one dinner roll) it takes me weeks for the symptoms to cease. Consequently, I now avoid gluten at all costs.

GETTING INTO THE GUTS OF NON-COELIAC GLUTEN SENSITIVITY

Now that I have gotten the stodgy stuff out of the way, I want to shift your train of thought to a couple of possibilities that scientists believe could be contributing to the recent surge of people with NCGS. Keep in mind that I am not an expert in this field, and nor do I claim to be. My expertise is on my own body, and how it responds to the 13 food intolerances I have. Non-coeliac gluten sensitivity happens to be one of them.

While navigating the many questions I had on wheat and its precarious love child gluten, I kept asking myself if something is in the wheat grain itself that wasn't there before. Turns out, my hunch was correct. Essentially, the wheat we eat today is not the same grain our ancestors would have used in their breads and other cereal-based foods. Traditional techniques used for creating a loaf of bread took a couple of days (whereas modern breadmaking will produce a freshly baked loaf in a matter of hours). Back then, the grains needed to go through a fermentation process before being baked into a sourdough-type loaf. Our ancestors discovered that fermenting grains like wheat naturally breaks down any toxins (fungus) and irritant proteins (gluten), which then makes grains healthier for us to eat. The human body thrives from fermented foods, which is why most people tend to feel less bloated after consuming bread that is made from sourdough.

Agricultural practices have come a long way when it comes to growing modern wheat. Science has taken selected genetic components from different wheat species and created a hybrid plant that produces more grain, has a higher gluten content, and is more resistant to disease and the environment it is grown in. Researchers have also linked the application of nitrogen-based fertilisers with increases in the production of gluten in wheat. Soil-borne diseases (fungus and viruses) and insects are still a problem for grain-producing plants, and wheat crops are on their kill list. However, some pesticides and herbicides have been shown to be associated with gastrointestinal problems and to increase the risk of developing coeliac disease and gluten sensitivities in some people.[35]

Is your mind blown yet? Mine sure was, once I dived into the rabbit hole of researching the associations between agricultural practices, gut bacteria and gluten sensitivities. I have only brushed the surface in this chapter and explained the basics. The good news is that the right people are asking the same questions: why are people becoming sensitive to gluten, and how can we fix it?

For a table outlining the levels of salicylates, amines and glutamates in common gluten-free products you may be considering, see appendix A.

CHAPTER 8

Looking out for preservatives and additives

AVOIDING PRESERVATIVES AND ADDITIVES THESE days is almost impossible. They are in everything – medications, cosmetics, food and personal care items. Every time you take a Panadol, wash your hair, or apply make-up you are introducing multiple additives and preservatives to your body. Any food product that comes in a package will have some sort of additive to prolong its shelf life, enhance its colour or flavour, and prevent nasty bacteria from growing and poisoning us.

Here in Australia, more people are becoming concerned about food safety and the quality of their food supply. In recent years, Australia has had several high-profile incidents of food safety and product recalls, which have increased concerns and questions from consumers. Consumers are becoming more conscious of checking food labels for additives, but there still seems to be some general confusion around preservatives and additives – including what they do and whether they are our friend or our enemy.

RETURNING TO MORE NATURAL FOOD

Urbanisation changed the way we needed to store and preserve food. Most of us do not have a big enough backyard (or apartment balcony) to sustain our own (and perhaps our family's) survival by growing seasonal fruit and vegetables. Nor can we venture into the 'urban jungle' with our trusty bow and arrow to hunt for protein. We depend on our supermarkets and local farmers' markets to provide us with fresh, edible food. Global urbanisation and public demand for a wider variety of food choices has made food preservation an essential process, because we (consumers) want a never-ending supply of out of season and exotic foods from around the world.

In recent years, however, the notion that 'food is medicine' has changed how people approach healthy living. More people are getting on board and embracing a healthier lifestyle, and many now associate food additives and preservatives with potentially harmful chemicals. With increased sensitivity and knowledge of the effect of added chemicals in food, we're seeing a growing trend for home preserving various fruits and vegetables. Natural food preservation and fermentation is also making a revival as more people aim to be more sustainable in their daily lives. Personally, I believe that people are becoming concerned about what chemicals they consume, and preserving and fermenting food ourselves not only reduces waste and provides health benefits, but also enables more control over what we put in our bodies.

The good news is that pressure is now also mounting for food manufacturers to avoid using chemical preservatives. Consumers are demanding natural alternatives, and manufacturers are listening. In recent years, global food manufacturing giants have invested in reworking their recipes to remove artificial colours, flavours and additives. A leading US hotdog manufacturer, for example, now declares their hotdog sausages (frankfurters) have no added nitrites or artificial preservatives. They're now using celery juice, which is a natural source of nitrite, in place of the chemical compound sodium nitrite.[36]

In other examples, scientists are looking into using bioactive compounds instead of chemical food preservatives. Edible coatings and food packaging materials made from plant, animal, and microorganisms are revolutionising the natural food preserving industry.[37] Amazingly, future food designer Chloé Rutzerveld has developed an edible ecosystem that looks like it belongs in a sci-fi movie. Her project, titled 'Edible Growth', focused on the 'potential use of additive manufacturing in food production'. Rutzerveld demonstrated how a 3D food printer could print multiple layers to create a honeycomb cage called the 'greenhouse'. The greenhouse structure contains multiple live organisms such as the seeds and spores of edible plants and mushrooms. Once printed, it can be placed on a sunny windowsill where the natural process of photosynthesis (the process that makes all plants grow) takes place, and within three to five days the plants and mushrooms are fully grown. Then you can eat the whole thing![38]

While these changes are positive, it could still be years before food manufacturers really move towards using more natural solutions in place of chemical preservatives. And although manufacturers are trying to move into more ethical and natural food preservation practices, the thought of what is already in our food at times frightens me. As it is, I am limited to what pre-packaged foods I can eat. I've also had to remove certain fresh foods from my diet due to the way they are being handled. The introduction of natural and ethical food preservation practices also may not make food intolerances easier. In fact, in some cases the natural alternative may still be something certain people are highly sensitive to. A case of watch this space.

Now let's take a more in-depth look at food additives and preservatives, and how they are used in our modern diet. You can use this information to identify which additives and preservatives to avoid, should you become sensitive.

ADDITIVES

The following table outlines the food additives commonly used in commercially produced foods.

Additive name	Additive use
Anti-caking agents	Stop ingredients from becoming lumpy
Antioxidants	Prevent food from going rancid or spoiling
Artificial sweeteners	Increase sweetness without increasing calories or kilojoules
Colours	Enhance and improve the appearance of food and drinks
Emulsifiers	Stop fats from clotting together
Flavours and flavour enhancers	Intensify flavour and/or aroma and improve palatability
Flour treatments	Increase the rising speed and improve the strength and workability of the dough
Foaming agents	Increase or decrease foam (bubbles)
Food acids	Sharpen flavours and act as a preservative
Glazing agents	Create a shiny polished look and provide a protective coating
Humectants	Add bulk, retain moisture and improve softness; used to stabilise and lengthen shelf life through moisture control
Mineral salts	Improve the texture and tenderness of food (including processed meats, unusually tender meat)
Preservatives	Stop bacteria, fungus and mould (to name a few) from forming and spoiling food
Stabilisers and firming agents	Increase shelf life
Thickeners and vegetable gums	Thicken and improve texture

Not all food additives are likely to cause an adverse reaction in sensitive people. Additives such as anti-caking agents, food acids, thickeners, sweeteners, gums, emulsifiers and bleaches are generally safe to eat.

And now for the not-so-fun stuff.

PRESERVATIVES

Preservatives are used to prevent food from spoiling due to bacteria, yeasts, moulds, fungus – anything that could potentially cause food poisoning or death. Their purpose is to prevent changes in colour, flavour and texture while maintaining freshness.

You will find some sort of preservative in any food item that is pre-packaged and/or processed, and especially in cured meats, pre-packaged fruit or vegetables (diced fresh or semi-fresh), and canned or jarred sauces and dressings.

The following sections outline the food preservatives that sensitive people, like me, will generally react to.

Sorbates

Sorbates are used to stop the growth of moulds, yeast and fungi. You will find food-grade sorbates in baked goods, canned fruits and vegetables, cheeses, dried meats and fruits, ice cream, soft drinks, wine and yoghurt. Sorbates are odourless and tasteless and are synthetically produced from a combination of sorbic acid and potassium hydroxide.

The following table outlines the variations of sorbates used in this process.

Sorbic acid (E200)	A preservative found in many foods, cosmetics and pharmaceuticals. In its natural state, sorbic acid originates from the berries of the rowan tree (*Sorbus aucuparia*). However, for commercial use, all sorbic acid (and its salts) are manufactured synthetically. Used in yogurts and other fermented dairy products, fruit salads, confectionary, lemonade, cheese, baked goods, wine and soups.

Sodium sorbate (E201)	The sodium salt of sorbic acid (E200), used as a preservative against fungus and yeasts. Used in the same range of products as sorbic acid.
Potassium sorbate (E202)	The potassium salt of sorbic acid (E200), widely used as a preservative in foods, drinks and personal care products. It is odourless and tasteless, and synthetically produced from sorbic acid and potassium hydroxide. Potassium sorbate prolongs the shelf life of foods by stopping the growth of mould, yeast and fungus.
Calcium sorbate (E203)	The calcium salt of sorbic acid (E200), used as a preservative against fungus and yeasts.

Benzoates

Benzoates are used in a variety of products not just limited to food. As a food preservative, they prevent bacteria, yeast and fungi growth. Benzoates are found in cold drinks, juices, vinegars, wines and salad dressings. Sodium benzoate does occur naturally in some fruits, such as apples and plums. To be used as a preservative, however (not its natural function), it is extracted and synthesised.

The following table outlines the variations of benzoates used.

Benzoic acid (E210)	Occurs naturally in various fruits, food barks and tea, but is mostly prepared synthetically for commercial use. Acts as a preservative and antioxidant in fruit products, soft drinks, salad dressing and pickled produce.
Sodium benzoate (E211) Potassium benzoate (E212) Calcium benzoate (E213)	Salts of benzoic acid, act as a preservative and antioxidant that inhibits the growth of mould, yeast and bacteria. Used in fruit products, juices, soft drinks, salad dressing, medications and pickled produce.
Benzoate esters (E216 & E218)	Act as a preservative mostly against yeasts and fungi (not as effective against bacteria).

Sulphites and sulphates

Sulphites and sulphates have a long history of being used as a food preservative, particularly in wine. Sulphites are naturally occurring minerals; however, the type of sulphite that is used in today's food preservation isn't. When used as an additive, sulphite will prevent the growth of bacteria, mould and fungus, and enhance food colour. Sulphites have become a popular preservative and you can find them in just about everything (and still particularly in wine). Personally, I am finding that my limited number of pre-packaged food items is dwindling all the time as more manufacturers are using sulphites as a preservative.

The variations of sulphites and sulphates used in this process are shown in the following table.

Sulphur dioxide (E220)	Used as a preservative in food (mostly fruit) and drink (wine) for its antimicrobial properties, prevents products from rotting. Mainly used in dried fruits and vegetables, soft drinks and wine.
Sodium sulphite (E221)	Salt of sulphur dioxide, used to prevent dried fruit from browning and discolouring.
Sodium bisulphite (E222) Sodium metabisulphite (E223) Potassium metabisulphite (E224)	Prevent oxidation, preserve food, and commonly used in home winemaking processes.
Potassium sulphate (E225)	Salt of sulphur dioxide, used to prevent dried fruit from browning and discolouring. It is also used for the production of caramel colour (E150d), used in many beverages.
Potassium bisulphite (E228)	Prevents oxidation, preserves food, and commonly used in home winemaking processes.

Most fresh prawns and other crustaceans are soaked in a sulphite solution on the boat at the time of the catch. This helps to keep 'black spots' from developing on their shells.

Nitrates and nitrites

Nitrates and nitrites are important plant nutrients that occur naturally in the fruit and vegetables that we eat. Amounts are generally low; however, leafy greens, such as celery, silver beets, lettuce and spinach, that are grown in hot houses and hydroponically will have higher levels.

As a food additive, chemically made nitrates and nitrites are added as a preservative in processed meats, to enhance colour and to prevent the growth of bacteria, mould and fungus. Nitrates and nitrites assist in developing the cured meat flavour. They prevent unpleasant odours and flavours and stop the meat from going rancid.

Potassium nitrite (E249) **Sodium nitrite (E250)** **Sodium nitrate (E251)** **Potassium nitrate (E252)**	Salts of nitrates and nitrites, used to enhance colour and a curing agent for meat and fish products, and prevent the growth of harmful bacteria and spoilage. Used in cured meats and fish, sausages, some cheeses, and canned foods that contain bacon, ham and sausages.

Propionates

Propionates are commonly used in bread and baked goods to prevent spoilage and mould growth. Propionic acid is also used to prevent mould on the surface of cheese and pre-packaged goods as a nutty flavouring agent. Propionic acid is used as a preservative for animal feed to prevent mould and bacteria growth because it is 'kinder' on their digestion.

Propionic acid (E280) **Sodium propionate (E281)** **Calcium propionate (E282)** **Potassium propionate (E283)**	Used to prevent the growth of mould in baked goods and flours.

| Cultured or fermented (wheat, dextrose, whey powder) | Any ingredients that are listed as 'cultured' or 'fermented' are labelled as a natural preservative. However, the natural bacterium *Propionibacterium freudenreichii* is used as part of a propionic acid fermentation to achieve the characteristics of a nutty flavour. |

ANTIOXIDANTS

In food, antioxidants are added to delay oxidation. Oxidation is the process whereby, once oxygen gets to food, it spoils. For example, if you left a slice of ham on the bench top, the longer it is out in the air the more it will become slimy, pungent, and eventually inedible. The same thing happens when you leave some sliced fruit uncovered – the cells exposed to the oxygen in the air turn brown.

Citric acid (E330)	A food acid that naturally comes from citrus fruit, used in various biscuits, jams, tinned fruits, cheese, alcoholic drinks, cakes, soft drinks and fermented meat products. It regulates the pH in jams and jellies.
Propyl gallate (E310) Octyl gallate (E311) Dodecyle gallate (E312) Tertiary-butylhydroquinone (E319)	Used to prevent the breakdown of fats in edible oils, margarines, lard and salad dressings.
Butylated hydroxyanisole (E320) Butylated hydroytoluene (E321)	Used to prevent the breakdown of fats in edible oils, margarines, chewing gums, fats, nuts and instant potato products. Petroleum by-product; prevents food from spoiling due to oxidation.

MINERAL SALTS

Some experts and specialists claim that mineral salts are not likely to cause a reaction and so are safe to eat. Personally, this is not the case. There are three mineral salts that I will never go near again, and I felt it important to include them in this section of the book.

'LIGHTLY MARINATED FOR TENDERNESS'

My husband cooked me a delicious baked chicken dinner and I commented on how tender and juicy the chicken was. To my horror, I woke the next morning looking like I had gone 10 rounds in a boxing ring. My eyes were a viscous red, watering, awfully sore to touch and almost swollen shut. I was quite puzzled as to why this had happened because I was eating exceptionally clean and had not had any reactions for some time. Remembering that the chicken dinner was unusually tender, I asked my husband what brand he bought and went back to the supermarket to see if it was the chicken that produced my symptoms. I discovered that the product had a tiny description (easily missed) that it was 'lightly marinated for tenderness'. Whatever it was marinated in was a clear substance because the chicken looked raw, all pinkish white. I flipped it over to see what was on the ingredients list and saw the combined mineral salts E450, E451 and E452. I tested this a second time and yep, boxing ring round two! So, I have now added mineral salts on my never-to-eat-again list.

The mineral salts I avoid are outlined in the following table.

Diphosphates (E450) **Triphosphates (E451)** **Polyphosphates (E452)**	Synthetically prepared emulsifiers, stabilisers and humectants, generally used to improve the quality and texture of meat products, bread, sausages and cheese products (cheese spread).

FLAVOUR ENHANCERS

Flavour enhancers are designed to bring flavourful life to processed foods that would otherwise be bland, boring and unappetising. Most flavour enhancers (such as MSG) do not have any taste of their own, but when combined with other tasty additives (such as powdered cheese, powdered onion or garlic, herbs and spices), they tend to pack a flavourful punch.

Flavour enhancers in some form (natural or artificial) are in everything that is processed. You will most likely encounter artificial enhancers in snack foods (crackers, flavoured chips/crisps), powdered soups, bottled sauces, vegetarian pre-prepared meals and instant noodles.

Flavour enhancers focus on the flavour element of *umami* (a Japanese term that means 'pleasant or savoury taste'). MSG is used all over the world, and it didn't take food manufacturers very long to work out that the key to great flavour lies in the seasoning.

Glutamate – MSG (E620) **Monosodium glutamate (E621)** **Potassium glutamate (E622)** **Calcium glutamate (E623)** **Ammonium glutamate (E624)** **Magnesium glutamate (E625)**	All artificial, used as a salt substitute and to enhance flavour. Produce an artificial umami savoury flavour and are often combined together.
Disodium guanylate (E627)	Used in many processed foods to generate a savoury, meaty or broth-like flavour (also known as artificial umami)
Disodium inosinate (E631)	Mostly used in combination with MSG (rarely used alone) to enhance flavour in condiments, and as salt substitutes for soups, sauces and snack foods.
Ribonucleotides (E635; **combined E627 & E631)**	Typically used in flavoured chips, instant noodles and party pies.

Hydrolysed vegetable protein	A processed flavouring made from vegetable proteins (maize meal, soybean meal or wheat gluten) that gives a meaty smell and taste.
Textured vegetable protein	A processed flavouring made from vegetable proteins (soy protein, soy flour, cotton seeds, wheat and oats) that gives a meaty smell and taste.

ARTIFICIAL FOOD COLOURS

Artificial colours are added to processed foods and beverages to make them more visually appealing to consumers. They are added to replace colour loss when exposed to environmental elements (light, air, moisture and heat) and to correct colour variations in processed food and beverages. Even though artificial colours have had a long history of affecting behavioural issues in children and some adults, Australia has one of the highest product counts of food containing artificial colours. Regulators have been unwilling to act and claim that artificial colours are 'safe', even though repeated studies have found that they can affect behaviour and learning.[39] [40]

The good news is that manufacturers have listened to consumers' demands for more natural ingredients and are now switching to natural plant-based high-intensity colours in place of their artificial relation.

Artificial colours are found in lollies/sweets, baked goods, dairy and cheese, jellies, and processed snacks, and the ones to watch out for are as follows:

- tartrazine (yellow) – FD&C Yellow 5 (E102)*
- quinoline yellow – D&C Yellow 10 (E104)^
- sunset or orange yellow – FD+C Yellow No 6 (E110)*
- azorubine/carmoisine (E122)#
- amaranth – FD+C Red No 2 (E123)^
- erythrosine – FD+C Red No 40 (E127)*
- allura red AC – FD+C Red No 3 (E129)*
- indigotine – FD+C Blue No 2 (E132)*

- brilliant blue FCF – FD+C Blue No2 (E133)*
- green S (E142)#
- brilliant black BN (E151)#
- carbon black – vegetable carbon (E153)^
- brown HT (E155)#.

Note that annatto orange-yellow (E160B) is a natural food colouring that is extracted from the achiote shrub. Because it is a natural food colourant, annatto is often used in place of artificial colours.

---

*   Permitted in AU, NZ, US, EU
^   Permitted in AU, NZ, EU; banned US
#   Permitted in AU, NZ, EU; no permission sought US

PART III

Coming back to basics

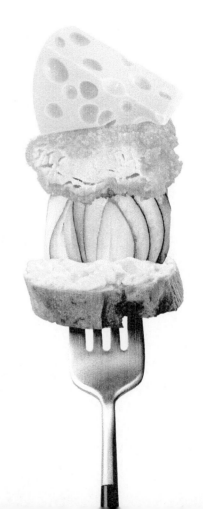

PART III

Coming back to basics

CHAPTER 9

Getting back to the basics of wellness

GETTING BACK TO BASICS IS *the* crucial aspect of managing any food intolerance. It's as simple as that. Most people already know the foundation to healthy eating, with it often being drummed into us from birth. Eat a variety of fruit, vegetables and legumes, whole grains, lean sources of protein (meat, poultry, seafood, nuts, legumes) and dairy. But how much is too much? And when it comes to food intolerances, any one of these food groups can become the enemy. This means going back to basics is the only way to return to a natural state of health.

A crucial factor to my food intolerance recovery and maintenance was to focus on my health in a holistic way. I've mentioned throughout this book that eating is not the only enemy and other lifestyle factors come into play. For me, the pathway to health and wellness was not just nutritional; I also needed to step into my body and take back control. This included focusing on my mind, body and spirit. Don't worry, I'm not going to go all woo-woo on you, but it is important to understand that a healthy body integrates with a healthy mind and spirit, and I had to wade through a lot of unhealthy conditioning to find my ideal balance.

This is how I did it!

EMBRACING MINDFULNESS AND MEDITATION

Outside of nutrition, a vital part of my road to recovery was through practising mindfulness and meditation. I needed to slow down, to work with my body and not against it. I'm a pretty busy person, working full-time, maintaining a family and household, studying and writing this book. Like most people, I have to constantly work on a healthy life–work balance.

Guided meditations are what keep me sane! They help me to stay present and to deal with any challenges thrown my way. When my nervous system is responding to stress or food sensitivities and I am feeling anxious, agitated and emotional, slipping into a guided meditation always calms me down. It helps me to relax, and become focused and in control of any uncomfortable bodily sensations I am experiencing.

Mindfulness is all about being fully present in my day-to-day life. It helps me not to become overly reactive or overwhelmed by what's going on around me. It brings awareness to what I am directly experiencing and helps me to stay on top of any physical and emotional reactions I have from my food sensitivities.

MINDFULLY EATING

Mindful eating is something else that I practice, and I find it to be very helpful with managing my food sensitivities. To me, mindful eating is all about being aware of the food I put into my body at all times. It's about being in tune with how my body is going to respond to the food that I eat and whether or not that response will be a healthy one.

For example, I cannot eat red tomatoes due to their salicylate and glutamate content, but I can eat yellow and orange ones. While this might seem weird, it's because the yellow and orange tomatoes have lower levels of salicylates and glutamate and I find that my body does not respond when I eat them. But I still have to be mindful of how much I eat. If I eat too many of them, then my body can become reactive and that's not ideal.

MANAGING DIGESTION AND NUTRITION

Healthy digestion is crucial when it comes to food intolerances. Knowing what works and what doesn't for your digestive system is indispensable for managing nutrition on a daily basis. I am mindful of how my gut is feeling all the time. For instance, I discovered that whenever I eat beef, it slows down my digestion, big time. It takes days for my body to fully process it and, during this time, I am more susceptible to becoming reactive if I am not careful with what I eat. This doesn't mean that I don't eat beef but, when I do, I am aware of how long my body takes to process it and plan ahead.

Managing nutrition is the only way you can stay on top of food intolerances. I cannot emphasise enough that it is imperative to know what your food sensitivities are before you can successfully manage them. Once you know, managing your nutrition is as simple as planning and being prepared. I am the only one in my household who has this affliction, and I am really lucky that my family support me. Our meals are planned around what I can and cannot eat and I like to aim for a variety in our meals because, let's face it, over time food intolerances can become bland and boring. I sure as hell do not want to eat food that is bland and boring, and neither does my family.

Food sensitivities rob the body of essential vitamins and minerals, and supplementation is an important aspect of food intolerance management. Once you have limited your intake of various foods and food groups, the micronutrients (vitamins and minerals) that the body needs to function are reduced. This can mess with your energy levels, your mental clarity and overall ability to function at an optimum level of health and wellness. I find that if I regularly miss my daily dose of supplements, everything (healthwise) goes down the drain. To stay on top of my health and support my immune system, supplements are a big part of my daily nutrition and wellness plan.

ADDING IN EXERCISE

Phew, we are almost there. I need to mention one more element that was an integral part of my food intolerance recovery: exercise. Exercise may be that dreaded thing you hate to do but try to do it anyhow, because you know it is good for you. There is a twist, however, and it was one that took me by surprise. My attitude towards exercise was always at the weight loss level – where you had to almost kill yourself, throw up or break something in order to feel like you have done a satisfying workout. I hated to exercise because of this and avoided it regularly. Not anymore. One of the things that food intolerance has taught me is to exercise smarter and not faster to get the results that I want. The key here is to find movement that you enjoy. I love to swim, ride my bike, walk my dog, and do yoga and reformer Pilates. All of these activities can be hard work, but because I enjoy them, I will do them regularly, which benefits me more than if I did a high-intensity aerobics class that I'd hate once a week.

You are now getting the picture that managing food intolerances is a never-ending balancing act. No one day is the same, but I guess that is the fun of having 13 food intolerances. I never get bored and there is always some form of challenge to take on to improve my prospects of leading a healthy yet flavourful life.

FOOD PREPARATION AND HOME COOKING

Eating a much higher proportion of homemade meals is how I took back nutritional control and conquered my food intolerance symptoms. Food intolerance is something I will have to manage for the rest of my life, but I believe that what worked for me can also work for you – and it's not as hard as it first may seem.

Simple home cooking is returning to the modern kitchen as more and more people are looking for alternatives to takeaway and highly processed meals. People with diets limited by food intolerances and digestive sensitivities will greatly benefit from switching to home-cooked meals in place of takeaway. Not only are home-cooked meals healthier for you, but they also allow greater control over the ingredients you use, and how the food is prepared. As an added bonus, the pleasures of sharing a home-cooked meal with your family and friends boost your confidence and self-esteem.

Finding the time and energy to prepare home-cooked meals can seem like a daunting task. At the end of a hectic day, the last thing you likely want to do is to spend another hour or two preparing the family meal. On top of the time restraints are the added stressors of cooking for someone with food intolerances and digestive sensitivities. Taking on this challenge is something I know my family avoids at all costs – cooking for my 13 food intolerances is a nightmare for them. But it doesn't have to be this way. Cooking with food intolerances and digestive sensitivities doesn't have to be as stressful or as complicated as it first seems.

Food preparation and home cooking is the reality of living with food intolerances and digestive sensitivities. It's something you can't avoid if you want to remain symptom free (or as close as possible to symptom free). Sure, it's great to eat out every now and then, and I'm not saying you can't, but getting back to the basics is what it takes to successfully manage food intolerances and digestive sensitivities. When it comes to nutrition for people with food intolerances, relying on what is easy, fast and convenient may no longer be an everyday option.

SHOPPING

My pantry is pretty light on pre-packaged food items and condiments. Most of my diet is based on fresh ingredients and even some of those I have to avoid because of their salicylate and glutamate content. I need to avoid almost all processed, pre-packaged foods due to the complexity of my food intolerances. And I still need to regularly monitor the limited pre-packaged food I do eat because manufacturers often change ingredients and additives to improve flavour and shelf life. This is why I cannot stress enough the importance of learning how to read labels. I know, standing in the middle of a supermarket aisle scanning ingredients lists is pretty tedious. It is a pain in the derriere trying to remember what all of those incomprehensible long words and numbers mean and whether or not you are intolerant to them. I provide some tips on quickly reading and understanding labels in the following section, but first let me give you a quick tip when doing your weekly grocery shop.

When visiting my local supermarket, I have learnt to 'shop the boundaries'. I find this really easy to remember because all of the food that I can eat is located around the edges of the store. Almost all supermarkets are laid out the same and you will find that they group their fresh ingredients together. This has cut my shopping time in half because I rarely have to navigate my way through all the aisles unless there is something in there that I need. When I do venture in, I have to be extremely picky with what I choose to buy. Label reading is a necessary part of my shopping experience, and I cannot express how important it is when it comes to successfully managing food intolerances.

Reading food labels

I know that label reading can be a tiresome, boring and confusing task, and you might be wondering why you should do it. Manufacturers are required to include warnings or advisory statements on products for foods that can be a health risk to some consumers, but that does not include warnings for people with food intolerances. It would be a labelling nightmare to put warnings or statements around the many different aspects of food intolerances and sensitivities. This is where understanding the ingredients list on a food label becomes a necessity.

But have you ever looked at a food label and wondered why you bothered? All of those long fancy words and numbers that mean nothing to you. Well, that is how I used to look at label reading – as far as I was concerned, what I didn't know couldn't hurt me, right?

Didn't I find out the hard way.

Now I will not buy anything that is pre-packaged or pre-cooked unless I know exactly what is in the ingredients. Being able to quickly work this out is a handy skill to have. I cannot tell you how many times I have picked up a product that I could previously eat, read the label and put it back because the manufacturer has made changes to the ingredients – it has saved me from a lot of physical pain from unexpected food intolerance reactions.

Food Standards Australia New Zealand (FSANZ) guidelines for food labelling have certain requirements. Any packaged food available for purchase in Australia must display the product's nutrition information, its ingredients, a list of food allergens (if applicable), the date for storage purposes, country of origin, health and nutrition claims (such as '98% fat free') and its Health Star Rating. The good news is that you don't have to know the ins and outs of all of these requirements. The only requirement I am interested in is the ingredients list.

To make this so much easier I am going take you through the ingredients list of a popular pre-packaged frozen food item – chicken tenders. Who doesn't love crumbed chicken?

Here's the ingredients list for a typical chicken tenders product:

Australian RSPCA Approved Chicken Breast (60%), Crumb [Maize Starch, Rice Flour, Tapioca Starch, Potato Starch, Acidity Regulators (Sodium Carbonates 575) Soy Flour, Dextrose, Yeast, Salt], Water, Canola Oil, Thickeners (1422, 1442, 412, 415), Rice Flour, Maize Flour, Salt, Egg Albumen, Soy Protein Isolate, Acidity Regulators (Sodium Carbonates, 541), Dehydrated Garlic, Dehydrated Onion, Mineral Salts (451, 450), Natural Colours (Turmeric, Paprika, Oleoresins) Pepper, Yeast Extract, Dextrose

These chicken tenders are quite tasty, and they were a rare go-to item I relied on when I was too tired to cook or wanted something fast and easy. You guessed it – I can no longer eat them because the manufacturer changed the ingredients and I started to react.

Here is why. The first ingredient listed is chicken. This particular chicken tenders recipe contains 60 per cent chicken – that is just over half of the listed ingredients. The other 40 per cent is various flours, starches, preservatives and powdered flavouring, which is where the fun begins.

Let's explore this a bit further. So, these particular chicken tenders are gluten and wheat free – which is indicated by the extensive list of various gluten- and wheat-free flours and starches (maze, rice, potato and tapioca). Most of the ingredients are standard, such as water, canola oil, salt and pepper, egg whites and baking soda. The ingredients I have to pay the most attention to are the dehydrated garlic and onion, mineral salts (451 and 450) and natural colours. These were the ingredients I reacted to that contained concentrated levels of salicylates and reactive preservatives (mineral salts).

Despite this being a complicated area, you do not have to be a science wiz to understand and read labels. To make shopping simpler, I now carry a wallet size list of food preservatives and additives code numbers that are likely to cause a reaction in me. I've provided this list in appendix D, or you can download a copy from my website (www.julieannwrightson.com).

CHAPTER 10

Getting back to the basics of flavour

WHEN I THINK ABOUT FLAVOUR, I get excited. That's because I am a food-lover, and love to cook and eat.

Prior to my food intolerance diagnosis, my analysis of my flavour palate was pretty simple – I either liked what I was eating or I didn't, and I never really considered why. Like most people, I followed recipes that someone else had designed. If I ventured out on my own and tried to 'reinvent' the recipe wheel, my resulting food creations were, quite frankly, disastrous. I even managed to turn one of my friends into a vegetarian after I tried to emulate a favourite chicken recipe my mum used to make. My food failures had that type of effect on the people around me. Consequently, my friends refused to eat when I tried to cook and went to great lengths to bring the point home, teasing me about their impending deaths from possible food poisoning and accompanying their assertions with dramatic demonstrations worthy of the last scenes of any Shakespearean tragedy.

FINDING PLEASURE IN FOOD – WITHOUT COMPROMISING MY HEALTH

Looking back, I can't blame my friends; my cooking was very creative, but not in a good way. I knew I was no MasterChef, but I didn't mind my own cooking so long as it tasted okay – I'd eat the overdone meat and sodden veggies.

Back then, I didn't really understand how recipes worked, or consider the fundamentals of flavour and how these aspects related to the meals I prepared. I was a self-taught cook, and it was blatantly obvious that I didn't know the first thing about technique and the chemistry involved in good cooking.

MY CULINARY ROOTS

As a small child I loved helping Nan in the kitchen – and I use the term 'helping' rather broadly. My idea of assistance was to lick clean the bowl and beaters after she had done all the hard work. I enjoyed being the taste-tester more than the creator and, as I got older, my culinary talents didn't improve much beyond that.

I relied on pre-packaged and pre-prepared food, or 'minimally prepared' food – where all I needed to do was to boil some pasta, noodles or rice, add cooked meat and veg, and throw in a jar of sauce. Dried or bottled sauces became a favourite because they were quick and easy and required little technical effort outside of boiling water, grilling, or opening a jar and adding heat.

Many years later, my food intolerance diagnosis forced me to change the way I eat. The specialists at the allergy unit taught me that, in most instances, the more flavoursome the food, the higher the chemical load – including salicylates, amines and glutamates – was likely to be. This means that when I added sauces, herbs, spices, salt rubs, coatings – anything that created flavour – I was likely increasing the natural and/or synthetic food chemicals and preservatives in the food I was eating. And I was adding these types of products to everything that I ate (or they were already present in the pre-prepared food I was buying). And it was what was making me sick.

My specialists recommended that when I cooked, I should keep my food plain, adding nothing flavour enhancing, except possibly salt and pepper. No sauces and, apparently, no flavour. Eating this way would keep my chemical load low and my body non-responsive, which was fantastic from a health perspective. But to eat this way forever felt like a death sentence. Flavour is what makes food palatable and enjoyable. To eat without flavour is like dining on cardboard – with a pinch of salt.

The allergy unit seemed to be condemning me to the daily drudgery of flavourless meal planning – I felt like I was trapped in a never-ending cycle of blandness and frustration. I was so bored of eating the same thing over, and over, and over again that food was no longer pleasurable. I was eating for the sake of survival and, quite frankly, this type of survival sucked. I was missing my favourite foods and I thought surely there had to be a way I could find pleasure with food again without compromising my health. Spoiler alert – there was. This is where a new chapter in my story started.

My journey to health and wellness has not been an easy one, and neither was my experimentation in the kitchen. Remember how my culinary skills were limited to turning people vegetarian and giving them possible food poisoning? Well, my food intolerance diagnosis forced me to expand (greatly!) the limited cooking techniques I knew. My unfortunate family became lab rats as I donned my mad scientist MasterChef hat and tried to create *flavourful* recipes from scratch. (Insert maniacal laugher and flickering lightning to the script at this point.)

Sometimes I succeeded and sometimes I didn't, but what my experimentation taught me was the fundamentals of flavour and how to use different ingredients to suit my palate and food intolerance needs. In the following sections, I share some ideas on how to bring flavour back to your food without overloading your chemical load and compromising your health.

THE ELEMENTS OF FLAVOUR

My best friend loves cheese. It doesn't matter what type she eats so long as it's cheese. My aunt puts tomato sauce on her peas and has for all the years I have known her. (Yuck, she used to make us eat it whenever we visited as children.) My husband loves chilli and anything that is hot and spicy (which is why he loves and married me, lol). I tend to lean towards the sweet/salty flavours that are prominent in Asian cuisines.

Flavour and taste are so very personal. Each of these examples shows the range of tastes even within the same family; however, what we all have in common is the link between flavour and an emotional response. I am sure that when you think about what you love to eat, certain memories and emotions are linked to this. And the memories and emotions we attach to certain foods and flavours are interesting and intense.

You experience the food you eat with your whole body, and not in a mechanical, processing way. I had always thought eating food was pretty mechanical – it went in your mouth, and your body processed it. If you didn't eat, you would die! But I now know there is so much more to eating than this simplistic approach.

Eating is more than just the basic instinct of survival. For some cultures, the art of taste is a way of life. Food tasting is constructed from the foundations of our five senses: taste, smell, sight, sound and touch. This is how I believe this works. I know that I am tempted to eat foods that look and smell fantastic. But what if I don't like the texture or how it feels in my mouth? Raw oysters are a great example. Some people love raw oysters. (Yay to you!) Me? I can't stand them. I hate how they feel in my mouth and when I try to swallow them. But I do enjoy oysters when they are cooked or smoked, so it's not so much about the taste but the texture of them that triggers my aversion. When you combine your taste senses like I did with the oyster scenario (texture and taste), you get an emotional response – and this is how we develop likes and dislikes to certain foods. We don't just eat in order to survive; we experience it.

Understanding flavour is vital when you are preparing food from scratch and managing food intolerances. You can then use natural flavours to your advantage. Adding flavour to food without compromising health is a skill that took me a long time to figure out and master. But that means you don't have to! I promise you that once you understand how flavour works and how to apply it to your cooking, eating will become pleasurable again, and cooking will be a joy.

THE FIVE FLAVOUR PROFILES

To truly understand how flavour works it is important to know about its basic profiles – sweetness, saltiness, bitterness, sourness and umami:

- **Sweetness** is sourced from foods such as sugar, honey, fruits and syrups. You likely know about the dangers of eating too much sugar, and I discuss the importance of not using artificial sweeteners in chapter 6. But the good news is that sugar is not completely the enemy, and using it in your cooking is essential because sweetness counteracts bitter and sour flavours. Ultimately, this helps balance the dish, our emotions and energy levels.

- **Saltiness** plays a couple of important roles in flavouring food. It enhances the other flavours in your dish, particularly sweetness. Think about that salty/sweet combination of things like salted caramel, sweet and salty popcorn, honey-soy. If your dish becomes too bitter, you can add salt to balance it out.

- **Bitterness** is what makes your face responsively scrunch up, and makes you stick your tongue in and out trying to rid your mouth of the taste (well, at least that's what I do). However, bitterness is an essential element in balancing flavour, and it gets those digestive juices flowing.

- **Sourness** involves further face-pulling and is great for enhancing one's cheekbones (as in, you pucker your mouth in response). A true sour taste for me feels like it causes the sides of my mouth to cave in. You will find sourness in vinegars, citrus and anything (cooking related) that is acidic. It's the acidity in the sour that balances your dish and brings liveliness, as well as counteracting sweetness and heat. I like to think of sourness as the Berocca of cooking, it gives your dish that b-b-bounce.

- Lastly is **umami**. I had no idea what umami was until I started to apply the elements of flavour to my cooking techniques. Umami is a complex taste profile that is embedded in the Japanese culture but has relevance to this subject. It is a Japanese term that translates as a 'pleasant, savoury taste' and is described as the full-bodied, meaty-type flavour of a dish.

I've discovered that you don't have to be a cuisine connoisseur to understand and apply umami to a meal. Once you do, you are enhancing its flavour by adding natural (or chemical) ingredients that contain glutamate (MSG) to complement the flavour. As I outline in chapter 5, glutamate occurs naturally in foods such as mushroom, seaweed, tomatoes and grapes. (See chapter 5 for a full list of foods that contain glutamate.) Glutamate in its chemical form is known as monosodium-glutamate or MSG and is used in Asian cuisines and pre-packaged food to enhance flavour.

What I didn't understand when I was experimenting with flavour was that I was unwittingly applying all five flavour elements in a very creative and unusual way. I was extracting flavour from my limited food list through various cooking methods and techniques. For example, there is a vast difference in flavour and texture between roasted and raw nuts. A raw nut has a fairly flat flavour and creamy texture compared to a crunchy, crisp roasted one.

ON THE ROAD TO FLAVOUR-TOWN

Once I made my mind up that I wasn't going to live a flavourless life, I started to watch cooking shows, especially Jamie Oliver's. He taught me how to go back to the basics of cooking and how to extract maximum flavour from my limited list of ingredients. Because of my previous culinary inventions, branching out on my own was a little scary. But I did it anyhow and I am so glad I worked up the courage to experiment with food again – and not cause food trauma in anyone during the process.

I found that if I added a bit of lemon zest to my chicken crumb (gluten free, of course) it put a bit of zing (sourness) back into the flavour. I experimented with other ingredients on my 'can eat' list, and now I have a crumbing mixture that is versatile and delicious – and, most importantly, doesn't overload my chemical threshold or compromise my health. (You can find this recipe in chapter 12.)

As my courage and knowledge grew, I became more adventurous and started to think further outside my limited culinary box. I started using ground nuts and dried legumes and vegetables to see if they would enhance flavour. I donned my 'Breaking Bad' hazmat suit and brewed impressive marinades and sauces that either intensified (or, worst case, dissolved) my protein of choice. The mad MasterChef was back and for a while there I felt a kindred connection with Heston Blumenthal, developing crazy concoctions and food combinations that should never have existed and defied the laws of classical food preparation. The more I experimented with my food, the more I thought about the fundamentals of flavour and how they worked or didn't work together.

I spent hours poring over old recipes, wondering if I could apply any of my new techniques to create a dish that could resemble the original, yet stay within the confines of my new eating rules. Mentally, I deconstructed their ingredients, using my imagination and memory of individual flavours. I thought about how each of the key ingredients in the recipe tasted and if I could replace it with something on my 'can eat' list. I pondered over the different styles of particular food cultures (such as Italian, Asian and Greek) I used to love, and wondered if I would be able to recreate their wonderful flavour combinations to suit my new dietary needs.

What surprised me most was the success I had in creating flavours that were pleasurable to a wide range of people. These flavours are not what would be considered classic Italian, nor are they purely Asian. What I have created is a unique taste blend that includes multiple food cultures and, most importantly, these flavours are food intolerance friendly. Jackpot!

THE FLAVOUR EFFECT

The practical application of cooking (in your day-to-day life of eating for survival and enjoyment) is being able to cook good flavourful food. Now let's consider the concept of 'layering' in cooking, and what I like to call the 'flavour effect'.

In my version of cooking (my family and I jokingly call it 'Julie-Ann's School of Culinary Arts') you can apply flavour layering, or the flavour effect, to your food in multiple ways. No hard or fast rules exist, and that is because we are all individuals with different tastes, different nutritional needs, and different sensitivities. Therefore, the 'recipes' in this book can be adjusted to allow for this level of self-management without impairing flavour too much. The beauty of the flavour effect is that flavour profiles can be added or removed based on your sensitivities, tastes and preferences, and taking into consideration your 'can eat' list.

The first level is the foundation of the recipe. The foundation ingredients are what make up the base of the recipe. For example, if you are going to make a flat bread that is flavoured with garlic and chives, the base or foundation of the recipe will be flour, salt, a liquid (water, milk, nut milk), a dash of sugar and oil. If you have the right ratios, these ingredients will make a quick and easy flat bread. If you are really sensitive or experiencing symptoms from a food intolerance reaction, you could stop here and have a tasty, low-chemical flat bread that can either be eaten on its own or as an accompaniment to other foods.

But I find plain flat bread flavoured only with salt and sugar becomes a bit tiresome after a while. Level two is where the fun begins and where I add or remove flavour to suit my taste and tolerance levels.

Continuing with the flat bread scenario, you could also add some finely grated (lactose-free) cheese, crushed fresh garlic and chives. The beauty of flavour layering (the flavour effect) is that you can pick and choose what you add or don't add to enhance the flavour of the flat bread. Personally, I can have all three of the added ingredients so long as the garlic and chives are fresh and not commercially dried or powdered. (I am fine when I dry my own and that is because I have more control over the freshness and concentration levels than if I bought it premade at the supermarket. Plus, I would not add any preservatives to prolong the shelf life.)

The third and final level is the technique or method of the recipe. The technique of a recipe is the details that tell you how to put the recipe together. It will include what equipment you need, how to combine and cook the ingredients (such as kneading dough or baking in an oven), and the length of time it takes for the recipe to cook. Famous American chef and author Julia Child called this a 'battle plan'. The good news is that the recipes I have created are easy to follow with basic cooking techniques, so you don't need to be a MasterChef to use them (or prepare for battle).

Now, this is where the fun part begins. Plug in your appliances, grab your mixing bowls, raise your wooden spoons – and get ready to cook!

CHAPTER 11

The food intolerance friendly pantry

A WELL-STOCKED PANTRY MAKES IT easier to prepare food intolerance friendly meals that align with your specific dietary needs. Your pantry can include a variety of whole, nutritious and minimally processed ingredients, which align with your desire for more natural and nutrient-dense options.

The foundation layer of your pantry stocks should be the basics. The rule here is to stock your pantry mostly with food items that you are confident using and that you love to cook with and eat. I've provided here a list of ingredients that I keep in my food intolerance friendly pantry. These ingredients are the bare bones of my cooking and I have them on hand always. I guarantee you will turn to these ingredients again and again when you begin to build your own food intolerance friendly pantry.

Consider stocking your pantry with the following:

- **Gluten-free flours, starches and baking needs:** Plain (all-purpose) flour, self-rising flour, almond flour, coconut flour, arrowroot flour, brown and white rice flour, cassava flour, tapioca starch, cornflour starch, baking soda, baking powder, vanilla essence, cacao powder, dark chocolate chips and xanthan gum.

- **Gluten-free grains:** Quinoa (grains, puffed and flakes), rice (any kind).
- **Herbs and spices:** This one is a bit tricky. I would suggest you keep either dried or fresh herbs and spices that adhere to your food intolerance nutrition plan. For instance, my herb and spice list is very small and consists of garlic, ginger, parsley, chives, coriander, coriander seeds, pepper, salt and bay leaves.
- **Sweeteners:** Brown sugar, natural sugar, maple syrup, rice bran syrup, honey (if tolerated).
- **Oils and vinegars:** Extra virgin olive oil, grapeseed oil, canola oil, rice bran oil and sesame oil. Malt vinegar, rice wine vinegar and apple cider vinegar.
- **Nuts:** Cashews, almonds, walnuts, peanuts, pecans, pine nuts, pistachios and macadamia. (I generally buy my nuts raw and unsalted.)
- **Legumes:** Canned or dried without any flavouring or sauces (chickpeas, white beans, black beans, four bean mix, kidney beans).
- **Dried products:** Good-quality gluten-free dried pasta, rice noodles, rice paper.
- **Condiments and spreads:** Peanut butter (smooth and crunchy), Bragg's Liquid Aminos All Purpose Seasoning (soy protein or coconut). Soy sauce substitute, good quality mayonnaise.
- **Fridge – dairy substitutes, lactose-free and dairy-free options:** Nuttelex (dairy-free margarine spread), lactose-free cheese, lactose-free yogurt or coconut yogurt, lactose-free milk or milk alternative (almond, macadamia).
- **Freezer:** Frozen berries, bananas and vegetables, chicken pieces (breast, thighs, wings, legs), beef and lamb. (I am not a big seafood person, and you will rarely see me eating it. I do like salmon and barramundi, calamari and prawns, in moderation. If seafood is what you love, then by all means fill your fridge or freezer.)

- **Fruit and vegetables:** As with herbs and spices, fruit and vegetables can be a bit tricky for some people. The basics that I keep in my fridge are apples, oranges, lemons, lettuce, cucumbers, avocado, zucchini, shallots, spring onions, snow peas, fresh beans, blueberries, raspberries, orange or yellow tomatoes, leek, potatoes, sweet potatoes and pumpkin.

Remember, the key to creating a food intolerance friendly pantry is to make sure the food items you choose are minimally processed, mostly fresh, and include ingredients that support your cooking ability, lifestyle and nutritional needs.

COOKING TOOLS, UTENSILS AND APPLIANCES

You really do not need a lot of fancy equipment or tools to create delicious food. The following list covers the essential cooking items you need when preparing and cooking family meals:

- **Cookware:** Frying pan, saucepans with lids (various sizes), stockpot with lid, baking trays, roasting pan, muffin trays, cake pans, pie dish.
- **Utensils:** Chef's knives, cutting boards, mixing bowls, mixing spoons, ladles, tongs, whisk, grater, can opener, peeler, rolling pin.
- **Food prep and cooking tools:** Measuring cups and spoons, colander/strainer, kitchen timer, thermometer (food/oven grade), kitchen scissors, meat tenderiser, kitchen scale, cooling racks.
- **Appliances:** Blender, microwave, food processor, toaster, electric kettle, handheld electric mixer.

Now that you understand the right ingredients, cooking tools and appliances, all you need now are the recipes.

CHAPTER 12

The recipes

A RECIPE IS THE BLUEPRINT that transforms a handful of plain and ordinary ingredients into something delicious. At its core, a recipe is a structured set of instructions that guides you through the process of cooking or baking a particular dish. It serves as a roadmap, detailing the ingredients, quantities, preparation steps and cooking techniques that are needed to create a specific meal or dish.

Recipes are not just a set of instructions, however; they also a gateway to the world of flavours, textures and culinary creativity. Getting back to the basics of recipes will empower you to embark on a flavourful journey through the world of cooking. It will unlock the secrets to food intolerance friendly food, and help you create satisfying and delectable meals.

STOCK AND SOUP

I like to use homemade liquid stock to enhance the flavour of my food. It provides a strong, intense flavour and adds depth and complexity to soups, stews, sauces, gravies, risottos and other dishes. I like to have three versions of stock on hand – chicken, beef and vegetable – to use as a quick and versatile solution for adding a savoury base to the dishes I cook.

The following recipes yield around 2 litres of stock concentrate per option. I divide the stock into one- and two-cup lots. I then freeze these portions – either creating frozen bars from a silicon mould that holds approximately one cup per bar or using a square plastic container that holds two cups. For smaller portions, I freeze the stock in square ice cube trays. Once frozen, I remove the stock from the moulds and store in an airtight container or zip lock bags.

Rich beef stock

- Moderate chemical load: contains amines and salicylates
- Free from egg, gluten, dairy, nut and soy
- FODMAP friendly: substitute spring onions with some chives or only use the green tops of the spring onion
- Prep time: 15 minutes
- Cooking time: 1 hour oven plus 8 hours stove top or 8–10 hours slow cooker
- Makes about 10 cups

Ingredients

- 2.5 kilos beef bones – include some osso buco beef cuts for flavour and richness
- Olive oil (for roasting)
- 3–4 litres of water
- 1–2 large carrots, cut in half
- 1–2 spring onions, peeled and cut in half
- 1 celery stem, cut in large chunks and including the leaves
- ½ tbsp coriander seeds (if tolerated)
- ½ tbsp pepper corns

- 1 tbsp apple cider vinegar
- 2 bay leaves (if tolerated)
- Small bunch of parsley, including stems

Method

1. To roast the bones, preheat oven to 200 °C/390 °F.

2. Add a splash of olive oil to two baking trays and spread bones over trays.

3. Roast the bones for 1 hour, turning them after 30 minutes, or until browned.

4. Place the bones in a large 5–7 litre capacity pot.

5. Drain any excess oil in baking tray and place the tray on the stove with ¾ cup of water to deglaze. Once the tray is simmering, start scraping the dripping from the tray to loosen and dissolve. Once the drippings are removed from the bottom of the tray, scrape all of the liquid into the pot. Repeat with the other tray.

6. Add the water to the pot, pushing the bones down to fit. Add more water if needed.

7. Add all remaining ingredients into the pot.

8. Bring the pot to the boil on medium-high and then turn down to low and gently simmer.

9. Simmer for 8 hours on very low heat with no lid. If using a slow cooker, cook for 8–10 hours on low.

10. After cooking time is up, fish out the bones and pour stock through a fine mesh strainer into a large bowl. Leave the strainer for a few minutes to let all of the liquid drip into the bowl.

11. Cool stock to room temperature or put overnight in the fridge.

Chicken stock

- Low to moderate chemical load: contains amines and salicylates
- Free from egg, gluten, dairy, nut and soy
- FODMAP friendly: substitute spring onions with some chives or only use the green tops of the spring onion
- Prep time: 15 minutes
- Cooking time: 2–3 hours stove top
- Makes about 10 cups

Ingredients

- 2–4 chicken carcases or 3 kilos of chicken wings, or a combination of both
- Rock salt
- Olive oil (for frying)
- 3–4 litres of water
- 1–2 large carrots, cut in half
- 1–2 spring onions, peeled and cut in half
- 1 celery stem, cut in large chunks and including the leaves
- ½ tbsp coriander seeds (if tolerated)
- ½ tbsp pepper corns
- 1 tbsp apple cider vinegar
- Small bunch of parsley including stems

Method

1. Place chicken carcases and/or wing pieces in a large 5–7 litre pot. If using chicken wings, with a large sharp knife carefully cut the wings into pieces at the joints, creating three pieces. (Trust me, this makes a very tasty stock.)
2. Add a handful of rock salt and a splash of olive oil to the chicken pieces and cook over the stove on medium heat. Let the chicken pieces brown a bit, stirring so they don't stick to the bottom.
3. Once the chicken pieces are lightly browned, add the water and the rest of the ingredients.

4. Bring the pot to the boil on medium heat and then turn down to low and gently simmer.

5. Simmer for 2–3 hours on very low heat with no lid.

6. After cooking time is up, fish out the chicken pieces and pour stock through a fine mesh strainer into a large bowl. Leave the strainer over the bowl for a few minutes to let all of the liquid drip into the bowl.

7. Cool to room temperature or put overnight in the fridge.

Vegetable stock

- Low to moderate chemical load: contains amines and salicylates
- Free from egg, gluten, dairy, nut and soy
- FODMAP friendly: substitute spring onions with some chives or only use the green tops of the spring onion; do not add the garlic
- Prep time: 15 minutes
- Cooking time: 1–2 hours stove top
- Makes about 10 cups

Ingredients

- 2 tbs olive oil
- 6 celery stalks, chopped
- 3 carrots, chopped
- 1 parsnip, chopped
- 1 swede, chopped
- 1 clove garlic, roughly chopped
- 1 2cm cube ginger, roughly chopped
- Salt to taste
- 1 tbsp peppercorns
- 1 tbsp coriander seeds (optional, if tolerated)
- 4 litres water
- 1 can of chickpeas – or fresh chickpeas, soaked for at least 24 hours before use
- 3 bay leaves crushed
- Low chemical load herbs – for example, parsley, coriander, or herbs of your choice (ones you can tolerate)

Method

1. Add the olive oil and all the veggies, ginger and garlic to a large saucepan (5–7 litres will be big enough). Sauté over a low heat. Add salt, peppercorns and coriander seeds and sweat the ingredients until soft, stirring occasionally.
2. Once softened and fragrant, fill the pot with around 4 litres of water. Add the chickpeas, crushed bay leaves and other herbs of choice.

3. Cover and bring to a boil over a medium heat. Reduce to low and simmer for 1–2 hours.

4. Make sure you taste the stock while cooking.

5. Once you are satisfied with the depth of flavour, turn off the heat and leave the stock to cool before straining.

Feel-good chicken soup

- Low to moderate chemical load: contains amines and salicylates
- Free from egg, gluten, dairy, nut and soy
- FODMAP friendly: substitute spring onions with some chives or only use the green tops; do not add the garlic.
- Prep time: 15 minutes
- Cooking time: 30–45 minutes or until the veggies are cooked and tender
- Serves 4–6

Ingredients

- 1–2 tbsp olive oil
- 1 leek, chopped
- 1 cup celery, chopped
- 1 cup carrots, chopped
- 1 garlic clove, crushed
- 1 tbsp fresh ginger, grated
- 4–6 cups chicken stock
- Salt and pepper to taste
- 2 bay leaves
- 4 chicken breasts or boneless thighs
- 2 cups cooked quinoa or rice noodles or rice
- Lemon juice to taste
- Fresh herbs of your choice

Method

1. Heat oil in a big pot over stove top on medium heat. Add the leek, celery, carrots, garlic and ginger and sauté for around 3–4 minutes. Lower the heat to medium-low.

2. Add the chicken stock, salt, pepper and bay leaves and bring to a boil. Cover the pot and lower heat to a gentle simmer, for around 20 minutes.

3. Meanwhile, cook the chicken in a frypan until brown and cooked through. Shred or dice and set aside.

4. Prepare and cook the quinoa/rice/rice noodles as per packet instructions. Set aside.

5. Once the veggies and broth are cooked (veggies are soft with a bit of firmness), turn off the heat and set aside.

6. In individual serving bowls, place ½ cup of cooked quinoa/rice/rice noodles.

7. Add the shredded/diced chicken and ladle broth and veggies into the bowl.

8. Add a squeeze of lemon to each bowl.

9. Garnish with fresh herbs of your choice.

PASTRY AND FLAT BREAD

Potato-based pastry

- Low chemical load
- Free from gluten, dairy, nut and soy
- FODMAP friendly
- Prep time: approximately 1 hour

Ingredients

- 600 g potatoes, peeled and chopped
- 2 tbsp olive oil
- 2 cups (300 g) gluten-free self-raising flour
- 1 tsp gluten-free baking powder
- 1 tsp ground salt
- 1 beaten egg, or equivalent egg replacement

Method

1. Place potatoes in a saucepan over medium to high heat and boil until soft and mashable. (You don't want them soggy, just soft enough for a light fluffy mash.)
2. Drain cooked potatoes and mash using a sieve or a steel potato ricer. Set aside to cool a little.
3. Combine 2 cups of the finely mashed potato and the olive oil in a large bowl. Sift in the gluten-free self-raising flour and baking powder, and add the salt and beaten egg (or egg replacement) to the bowl.
4. Mix until it all comes together, adding extra beaten egg mixture as needed.
5. Lightly flour a large board to turn mixture onto, and knead until you get a smooth, silky dough.
6. Set aside in a clean bowl covered with a damp tea towel to keep the pastry light and moist.

Note: This pastry base is best used on the day of making or one day after. If storing overnight, store in an airtight container in the fridge. Uncooked pastry is not suitable for freezing.

Basic flat bread

- Moderate chemical load: contains amines
- Free from eggs, lactose, gluten, nut and soy
- Dairy-free alternatives can be used (as noted)
- FODMAP friendly when using lactose-free yogurt
- Prep time: 5 minutes
- Cooking time: 5 minutes or until any veggies are cooked and tender
- Serves 4–6

Ingredients

- 1 cup full-fat or lactose-free or dairy-free Greek yogurt
- 2 cups gluten-free plain flour blend, plus more for flouring, or a pre-mixed gluten-free bread blend (you can use regular flour or flour bread blend if not gluten sensitive)
- 2 tsp gluten-free baking powder (omit if using a pre-mixed bread blend)
- Salt, to taste

Method

1. In a large bowl, add the yogurt, gluten-free flour blend and baking powder (or bread blend), and salt. Mix until a dough forms.
2. On a lightly floured surface, transfer the dough and flatten into an 8-inch (20 cm) disk.
3. Cut 4 equal parts and flatten each part to your desired thickness. (I like mine around 6 mm thick, but you might like a thicker flat bread.)
4. Carefully transfer the dough pieces one at a time into a preheated non-stick pan, over medium heat.
5. Cook the first side until you see some bubbling, and then flip until well browned.
6. Serve.

Note: Before mixing the dough, you can add some additional ingredients for tasty variations:

- Add garlic and parsley for a garlic flat bread.
- Add finely grated cheese and some finely chopped chives.
- Add white and black sesame seeds for a nuttier flavour.

The options are endless!

SAVOURY DISHES

Food intolerance friendly tacos

- Moderate to high chemical load: contains salicylates, amines, glutamate
- Free from eggs, lactose, gluten and nuts
- Dairy-free alternatives can be used (as noted)
- FODMAP friendly: substitute spring onions with some chives or only use the green tops; do not add the garlic
- Prep time: 5–10 minutes
- Cooking time: 30 minutes
- Serves 4

Ingredients

- Olive oil (for frying)
- 500 g lamb or beef mince
- 2 small spring onions, diced
- 1 clove garlic, crushed (if tolerated)
- 2–3 cups of rich beef stock *(see recipe page 106)*
- 1 tbsp soy sauce or soy sauce substitute
- Salt and pepper to taste
- Taco shells – soft or hard (gluten-free options are available at the supermarket)
- 2 cups lettuce, thinly sliced
- 1 avocado, thinly sliced
- 1 cup grated cheese (lactose-free or vegan options are available at the supermarket)
- 1 large tomato or 5–10 orange or yellow cherry tomatoes thinly sliced (orange and yellow tomatoes are lower in salicylates and glutamate)

Method

1. Heat the olive oil in a large frypan with high sides, add the mince, spring onions and garlic and pan fry until the mince is starting to brown. Add the rich beef stock, soy sauce (or replacement) and salt and pepper to taste.

2. Reduce the heat and let the mince and stock simmer on low until all of the stock sauce has dissolved – approximately 10–15 minutes.
3. Prepare taco shells (soft or hard) as per packet instructions and arrange on a separate plate.
4. Arrange lettuce, avocado, cheese and tomatoes on a large board.
5. Place the cooked mince into a bowl and set near the board with the other ingredients.
6. To assemble the tacos, grab a taco shell and layer the other ingredients to taste.

Mushroom risotto

- Moderate chemical load: contains salicylates, amines, glutamate
- Free from eggs, lactose, gluten, nut and soy
- Dairy-free alternatives can be used (as noted)
- FODMAP friendly: substitute spring onions with some chives or only use the green tops
- Prep time: 5–10 minutes
- Cooking time: 30 minutes
- Serves 4

Ingredients

- 6 cups vegetable stock *(see recipe page 110)*
- 3 tbsp butter (or Nuttelex or lactose-free alternative)
- 2 garlic cloves, minced
- 2 small spring onion bulbs, sliced
- 2 cups button mushrooms, sliced
- Freshly ground black pepper
- Salt to taste
- 1½ tsp apple cider vinegar
- 1½ cups arborio rice
- ½ to ¾ cup shredded parmesan cheese (or lactose-free equivalent)
- Finely chopped fresh parsley, for garnish (optional)

Method

1. Warm the stock in a saucepan over medium-low heat. Make sure it does not boil.
2. In a large, high-walled frypan, heat the butter (or Nuttelex or lactose-free alternative). Add the garlic, spring onions, mushrooms, salt and pepper, and sauté over a medium to high heat until the onions begin to soften. Add the apple cider vinegar and cook until the mushrooms are soft and have darkened in colour. Transfer to a plate and set aside.
3. In the same saucepan, add the rice and stir for up to a minute. Add ¾ cup of the warm stock into the pan with the rice and stir. Reduce the heat to medium and stir, letting all of the liquid absorb.

Keep adding the stock ¾ of a cup at a time, stirring regularly until most of the stock has been absorbed by the rice – around 25 minutes. The rice should have a creamy consistency and still be a little wet.

4. Remove the frypan from the heat, stir in the mushroom mixture and parmesan cheese (or lactose-free equivalent).

5. Divide into four bowls. Add the parsley for garnish and serve.

AUSSIE MEAT PIE

- Moderate chemical load: contains salicylates, amines, glutamate
- Free from eggs, lactose, gluten, nut and soy
- Dairy-free alternatives can be used (as noted)
- FODMAP friendly: substitute spring onions with some chives or only use the green tops
- Prep time: 5–10 minutes
- Cooking time: 30 minutes
- Serves 4–6

Ingredients

Filling:

- 1 kilo beef or lamb mince (or 500 g of each combined)
- 2 spring onions finely chopped.
- 2–3 cups rich beef stock *(see recipe page 106)*
- 1 tbsp of soy sauce or soy sauce substitute (or to taste)
- Salt and pepper to taste
- 3 tbsp gluten-free flour
- ¼ cup water

Pie base:

- 1 serve potato-based pastry *(see recipe page 114)*
- 1 egg, beaten, or dairy-free butter/margarine (for glazing)

Method

Filling:

1. In a large frypan, combine the beef and/or lamb mince and spring onions and cook for 2 minutes on a medium to high stove top heat.
2. Add the beef stock, Coconut Liquid Aminos, salt and pepper and bring to a light boil.
3. Reduce the heat and let the mixture simmer for around 15 minutes, checking every five minutes or so to make sure that not all of the stock has been reduced and absorbed. (If mixture gets too thick, add a small amount of water.)

4. Blend the gluten-free flour with the water to make a slurry (thickish paste) and gently stir through until the mince filling has thickened.

5. Put aside to cool.

Pie base:

1. Pre-heat oven to 180 °C/350 °F.

2. Divide the pastry ball in half.

3. Lightly grease a family-sized pie dish.

4. Take half of the pastry and roll it out to the size of your dish. Line the dish with the bottom layer of the pastry, gently pressing the bottom and sides until the sides of the pastry come up and slightly over the top of your dish. This will help to create a good seal once you cap the pie filling.

5. Over the top of the pastry-lined dish, place some baking paper and 1 cup of uncooked rice. Spread the rice evenly around the bottom of the pie dish and put it in the oven to blind bake for 5–7 minutes. This step helps to prevent bubbles from forming in the pie shell.

6. Remove the pie shell from the oven and discard the baking paper and rice.

7. Increase the heat of the oven to 190 °C/375 °F.

8. Fill the pie base shell with the cooled mince mixture, spreading evenly.

9. Roll out the second ball of dough slightly larger than the pie dish and cap the pie.

10. Trim any excess pastry and pinch the edges together to seal.

11. Prick a few holes in the top with a fork and use the egg wash or melted butter/margarine to glaze the top.

12. Bake in the oven for 15 minutes or until the pastry is crispy and slightly browned.

13. Remove from the oven, cut and serve.

Basic quiche, family size

- Moderate to high chemical load: contains salicylates, amines, glutamate
- Free from eggs, lactose, gluten, nut and soy
- Dairy-free alternatives can be used (as noted)
- FODMAP friendly: substitute spring onions with some chives or only use the green tops; do not add the garlic
- Prep time: 5–10 minutes
- Cooking time: 45–60 minutes
- Serves 4

Ingredients

Filling:

- 4 eggs
- 2 tbsp butter or dairy-free alternative, melted
- 1 cup milk or milk alternative (I use almond milk)
- Squeeze of lemon juice
- 1 clove garlic, minced (optional)
- ½ tsp baking powder
- ¼ cup gluten-free flour to thicken
- Salt and pepper to taste
- Fresh chopped parsley/chives

Pastry base:

1 serve potato-based pastry *(see recipe page 114)*

Method

Pastry base:

1. Pre-heat oven to 180 °C/350 °F
2. Divide the pastry ball in half.
3. Lightly grease a family-sized quiche dish.
4. Take half of the pastry and roll it out to the size of your dish. Line the dish with the bottom layer of the pastry, gently pressing the bottom and sides until the sides of the pastry come up even

with the top of your dish. (You can use the other half of the pastry for another dish.)

5. Over the top of the pastry-lined dish, place some baking paper and 1 cup of uncooked rice. Spread the rice evenly around the bottom of the pie dish and put it in the oven to blind bake for 5–7 minutes. This step helps to prevent bubbles from forming in the quiche shell.

6. Remove the shell from the oven and discard the baking paper and rice.

7. Set aside and prepare the filling.

Filling:

1. In a mixing bowl, whisk together all of the filling ingredients until no lumps remain.

2. Pour the egg mixture over the crust.

3. Bake for around 40-45 minutes until the centre is set and no longer jiggles.

4. Allow the quiche to cool a little before eating.

5. Serve hot or cold.

Note: You can add ingredients to make this even tastier:

- Mushrooms: pre-cook in butter/dairy-free alternative and stir through the egg mixture before baking.
- Leek: pre-cook in butter/dairy-free alternative and stir through the egg mixture before baking.
- Cheese: stir any cheese you like through the egg mixture before baking.
- Bacon/ham: pre-cook and stir through the egg mixture before baking.

Potato gnocchi

- Low chemical load
- Free from gluten, dairy, nut and soy
- FODMAP friendly
- Prep and cooking time: approximately 1 hour

Ingredients

1 serve potato-based pastry *(see recipe page 114)*

Method

1. Lightly flour a large board and divide the potato dough into four equal portions.
2. Roll 1 portion of the dough into a 2-centimetre log reaching about 30 centimetres in length. Using a floured knife, cut into 2-centimetre pieces. Repeat with the remaining three portions.
3. For a more authentic-looking gnocchi, lightly flour your hands and roll each piece of dough into a ball. Use your thumb to roll each ball over a floured fork, and place on a tray. Repeat until all of the dough has been rolled and forked.
4. Over medium heat, bring a saucepan of salted water to a boil, add a quarter of the gnocchi and cook for three minutes. Do not overcrowd the gnocchi; otherwise, they will stick together.
5. Use a slotted spoon to scoop out the cooked gnocchi, making sure the water has drained. Place in a bowl and repeat until all of the gnocchi is cooked.
6. Add the cooked gnocchi to your favourite sauce.

Note: You can serve this gnocchi with your preferred sauce:

- For a tomato-based sauce, see the recipe for a basic orange tomato sauce on *page 131*.
- For a creamy sauce, see the basic creamy sauce recipe on *page 129*.

SAUCES, SALAD DRESSINGS AND MARINADES

Basic gravy – without drippings

- Moderate chemical load: contains salicylates, amines, glutamate
- Free from eggs, lactose, gluten, nut and soy
- Dairy-free alternatives can be used (as noted)
- FODMAP friendly: substitute spring onions with some chives or only use the green tops
- Prep and cooking time: 5 minutes
- Makes approximately 1½ cups

Ingredients

- 30 g butter (or dairy-free alternative)
- 1–2 spring onions or 1–2 French shallots, finely chopped (optional, if tolerated)
- 1½ tbsp plain gluten-free flour
- 1½ cups rich beef stock *(see recipe page 106)*
- Salt and pepper to taste
- Small handful of fresh finely chopped parsley or herbs of choice (optional, if tolerated)

Method

1. Melt the butter/dairy-free alternative in a large saucepan over a medium heat.
2. Cook the spring onions/French shallots and garlic, stirring for around 5 minutes or until browned.
3. Stir in the flour to coat the spring onions/French shallots and cook for around 30 seconds.
4. Slowly stir in the stock until well combined, making sure all of the brown bits are covered.
5. Bring the liquid to a boil and then reduce the heat. Gently simmer for around 4 minutes or until the sauce thickens. Stir occasionally so gravy does not stick to the bottom of the saucepan. Add in salt and pepper to taste.
6. For a smooth gravy, strain into a small jug. For a chunkier gravy, do not strain before transferring into a small jug. Stir in some chopped parsley to taste.

Basic gravy – with drippings

I like to make gravy from the leftover drippings from a baked dinner or anything I have cooked that has created crusty bits stuck to the pan. (Lamb meatball dripping makes a delicious flavoursome gravy.)

- Moderate to high chemical load: contains salicylates, amines, glutamate
- Free from eggs, lactose, gluten, nut and soy
- Dairy-free alternatives can be used (as noted)
- FODMAP friendly: substitute spring onions with some chives or only use the green tops
- Prep and cooking time: 5 minutes

Ingredients

- 30 g butter (or dairy-free alternative)
- 1–2 spring onions or 1–2 French shallots, finely chopped (optional, if tolerated)
- Up to ¼ cup of plain gluten-free flour
- 2 cups rich beef stock *(see recipe page 106)*
- Drippings from leftover baked dinner or pan fried meat/food. *Note:* If a lot of dripping liquid is left over from a baked dinner, strain into a bowl and add around 1 cup or to taste.
- Salt and pepper to taste
- Small handful of fresh finely chopped parsley or herbs of choice (optional, if tolerated)

Method

1. Melt the butter/dairy-free alternative in a large saucepan over a medium heat.
2. Cook the spring onions/French shallots and garlic, stirring for around 5 minutes or until browned.
3. Stir in the flour to coat the spring onions/French shallots and cook for around 30 seconds.
4. Slowly add the stock and drippings and whisk vigorously until fully heated through.

5. Add salt and pepper to taste and continue to heat for around 5 to 10 minutes or until the gravy has reached the desired thickness.

   Note: If the gravy is too thin, create a flour slurry by adding 1 to 2 tablespoons of gluten-free plain flour to a jar with a lid. Fill with water and shake until a thick sludge is formed. Gently and slowly add the slurry to the gravy bit by bit, whisking vigorously so it does not form lumps. If gravy is too thick, slowly add more stock or water until you get your desired consistency.

6. For a smooth gravy, strain into a small jug. For a chunkier gravy, do not strain before transferring into a small jug. Stir in some chopped parsley to taste.

Basic creamy sauce

- Low to moderate chemical load: contains salicylates, amines, glutamate
- Free from eggs, lactose, gluten, nut and soy
- Dairy-free alternatives can be used (as noted)
- FODMAP friendly: do not add the garlic
- Prep and cooking time: 10–15 minutes
- Makes approximately 2 cups

Ingredients

- 2 tbsp butter (or dairy-free alternative)
- 1 clove garlic, minced (optional)
- 1 cup chicken or vegetable stock *(see recipes pages 108 and 110)*
- 1 cup milk or milk alternative (I use almond milk)
- Gluten-free flour (to thicken)
- Squeeze of lemon juice
- Salt and pepper to taste
- Fresh chopped parsley/chives for garnish

Method

1. Melt the butter/dairy-free alternative in a large saucepan over a medium heat.
2. Add the minced garlic, if using, stirring to prevent burning.
3. Add the chicken or vegetable stock and the milk or milk alternative and bring to a boil.
4. Reduce the heat to a simmer.
5. Make a gluten-free flour slurry – see following instructions.
6. Gently and slowly add the slurry bit by bit, whisking vigorously so it does not form lumps.
7. Once the sauce has thickened, add a squeeze of lemon juice, salt and pepper to taste and fresh herbs for garnish.

Make a flour slurry: Add 1 to 2 tablespoons of gluten-free plain flour to a jar with a lid. Fill with water/milk or milk alternative and shake until a thick sludge is formed.

Note: You can vary this basic sauce by adding mushrooms, cheese or herbs of your choice.

Sticky Asian-inspired sauce

- Moderate chemical load: contains salicylates, amines
- Free from eggs, lactose, gluten and nuts
- Dairy-free alternatives can be used (as noted)
- FODMAP friendly: do not add the garlic
- Prep and cooking time: 10–15 minutes

Ingredients

- 2 tsp sesame oil
- 1–2 tsp fresh ginger, minced
- 2 cloves garlic, minced
- 2 cups chicken or vegetable stock *(see recipe pages 108 and 110)*
- 2 tbsp rice vinegar
- ¼ cup brown rice syrup
- 2–4 tbsp soy sauce replacement or to taste
- 2 tbsp maltose (available at Asian supermarkets – this makes it 'sticky')
- Gluten-free plain flour (to thicken)

Method

1. Over a medium heat, add the sesame oil, ginger and garlic, and stir to prevent the garlic from burning.
2. Combine the stock, rice vinegar, brown rice syrup and soy sauce/ soy sauce replacement and add to the pan.
3. Bring the liquid to a boil and then reduce heat to a simmer.
4. Add the maltose and stir until it is fully dissolved.
5. Make a gluten-free flour slurry – see following instructions.
6. Gently and slowly add the slurry bit by bit, whisking vigorously so it does not form lumps.
7. Once the sauce has thickened and become 'sticky' it is ready to serve.

Make a flour slurry: Add 1 to 2 tablespoons of gluten-free plain flour to a jar with a lid. Fill with water/cold stock/milk or milk alternative and shake until a thick sludge is formed.

Basic orange tomato sauce

- Moderate to high chemical load: contains salicylates, amines
- Free from eggs, lactose, gluten and nuts
- Dairy-free alternatives can be used (as noted)
- FODMAP friendly: substitute spring onions with some chives or only use the green tops; do not add the garlic
- Prep and cooking time: 10–15 minutes
- Suitable to make in bulk; freezable

Ingredients
- 2 cups chicken stock *(see recipe page 108)*
- 3 punnets orange or yellow cherry tomatoes
- 1 large spring onion, diced
- 2–3 garlic cloves, crushed
- 1 tbsp plain gluten-free flour (for thickening)
- Fresh coriander or herb of choice, chopped (optional)
- Salt and pepper to taste

Method
1. In a medium to large saucepan, combine the chicken stock, tomatoes, spring onion and crushed garlic. Bring to a gentle boil.
2. Once boiling, reduce heat and simmer until the tomatoes, onion and garlic are soft and mashable.
3. With a hand blender, puree until smooth (or leave a bit chunky – however you like it).
4. If the sauce is a bit runny, add small amounts of gluten-free plain flour to thicken.
5. Add fresh herbs, salt and pepper to taste.

Note: If you are making this in bulk, do not add the fresh herbs before freezing. Add fresh herbs when you are reheating the defrosted sauce.

I use this sauce in place of a red tomato based pasta sauce. Add it to any type of pasta (including gluten-free options and the potato gnocchi on *page 125*). Add grounded meat of choice for a great tasting bolognaise or use it as a topping sauce for grilled chicken breast.

Cashew nut cream

- Low chemical load: contains salicylates, amines
- Free from eggs, lactose, gluten and soy
- Dairy-free alternatives can be used (as noted)
- Not suitable for FODMAPs
- Prep time: 4 hours
- Cooking time: 5–10 minutes

Ingredients

- 1 cup raw cashews (150 g)
- 1 tbsp lemon juice (optional)
- ½ cup water
- 1 tsp rice malt syrup (or to taste)
- Salt to taste

Method

1. Soak the cashews in water for around 2–4 hours.
2. Add the cashews with all other ingredients to a high-speed blender and blend until smooth.
3. Nut cream can be stored in the fridge for up to a week.

Sour cream alternative: Add 1 tsp of apple cider vinegar, ¼ tsp of Dijon mustard (optional, as tolerated) and blend until smooth.

Note: I like to use this in multiple ways. I have added it to cream-based recipes for added flavour, mixed it with some hummus and used it as the base sauce on a gluten-free pizza. I have topped apple wheels with a dollop of sweetened cashew nut cream and used the sour cream alternative to top roasted potatoes.

Low-chemical mayonnaise

- Low chemical load: contains salicylates, amines
- Free from lactose, gluten, soy and nuts
- Dairy-free
- FODMAP friendly
- Prep and cooking time: 10–15 minutes

Ingredients

2 egg yolks
¼ tsp salt, or to taste
1 cup neutral flavoured oil (grapeseed, safflower or canola go well)
1 teaspoon fresh lemon juice

Method

1. Place the egg yolks and salt in a bowl or blender and whisk/blend together until mixture thickens and is well combined.
2. Continue to whisk/blend and gradually add a quarter of the oil, bit by bit with a teaspoon. The mixture should become quite thick at this stage.
3. Still whisking/blending, slowly pour the remaining oil in a steady stream.
4. Once thickened, stir/blend in the lemon juice until well combined.

Note: Mayonnaise can be stored in the refrigerator for up to three days.

Sweet Asian-inspired salad dressing

- Low to moderate chemical load: contains salicylates, amines
- Free from eggs, lactose, gluten and nuts
- Dairy-free
- FODMAP friendly: do not add the garlic
- Prep and cooking time: 5 minutes

Ingredients

- 1 cup of grapeseed oil
- 1 tbsp of brown sugar, or to taste
- 1 tsp of rice wine vinegar
- 2 tbsp of soy sauce or soy sauce alternative
- Salt and pepper to taste
- 1 tsp fresh lemon juice
- 1 small garlic clove, crushed (optional)
- 1 small piece of ginger, grated (optional)

Method

1. Place all ingredients in a jar with a lid and shake vigorously until well combined. The dressing will thicken as the ingredients emulsify together.

2. Store in the fridge.

Note: When storing in the fridge, the dressing will separate. Bring it back to room temperature and shake to mix together.

Green goddess salad dressing

- Low chemical load: contains salicylates, amines
- Free from eggs, lactose, gluten, soy and nuts
- Dairy-free
- FODMAP friendly: substitute spring onions with some chives or only use the green tops
- Prep and cooking time: 5 minutes

Ingredients

- ½ large avocado
- ¼ cup parsley and/or coriander, including stems
- Juice of one lemon
- ⅓ cup grapeseed oil
- 2 garlic cloves, peeled
- 2 tbs low-chemical mayonnaise *(see recipe page 133)*
- 2 green spring onions, sliced (optional)
- ¼ to ½ cup water
- Salt and pepper to taste

Method

1. Place all ingredients and a ¼ cup of the water in a food processor and blend until all ingredients are well combined.
2. If the dressing is too thick, add more water until you get to the desired consistency.
3. Store in the fridge for up to a week.

Basic orange maple vinaigrette

- Low chemical load: contains salicylates, amines
- Free from eggs, lactose, gluten, soy and nuts
- Dairy-free
- FODMAP friendly
- Prep and cooking time: 5 minutes

Ingredients

- Juice of half an orange, or to taste
- 2 tbsp maple syrup, or to taste
- 2 tbsp apple cider vinegar
- ⅓ cup extra light olive oil
- Salt and pepper to taste

Method

1. Place all ingredients in a jar with a lid and shake vigorously until well mixed.
2. Store in the fridge for up to a week.

SOME OF MY FAVOURITE SNACKS AND DESERTS

Maple syrup glazed nuts

- Low chemical load: contains salicylates, amines
- Free from eggs, lactose, gluten and soy
- Dairy-free
- FODMAP friendly: do not add cashew and pistachio nuts to the nut mix
- Prep and cooking time: 20–25 minutes

Ingredients

- 1 tbsp olive oil
- ¼ cup maple syrup
- 1¼ cups almond kernels
- 1¼ cups pecans
- ¾ cup cashew nuts
- ¾ cup unsalted pistachio kernels
- ¾ cup macadamia nuts

Method

1. Preheat oven to 180 °C/350 °F and line a large baking tray with baking paper.
2. Whisk the oil and maple syrup together in a large bowl. Add nuts and toss to thoroughly coat.
3. Spread nuts onto prepared tray. Bake for 15 minutes, stirring halfway, or until golden.
4. Set aside to cool. The nuts will be soft while hot, but once cooked they will be lovely and crunchy.
5. Store in an air-tight container.

Basic vanilla chia seed pudding

- Low chemical load: contains salicylates, amines
- Free from eggs, lactose, gluten, soy and nuts
- Dairy-free
- FODMAP friendly
- Prep time: 5 minutes
- Three hours or overnight for setting

Ingredients

- ½ milk or lactose-free milk or dairy-free option (almond, cashew, oat or coconut milk)
- 2 tbsp chia seeds
- 2 tsp maple syrup, or to taste
- ½ tsp vanilla extract

Method

1. Mix all of the ingredients together in a Mason jar or bowl until combined.
2. Seal with a lid or cover and let sit in the fridge for a minimum of three hours; preferably overnight.
3. To serve, scoop out as much of the pudding as you wish and add toppings.

Toppings: Yoghurt (dairy-free if needed), fresh berries, sliced bananas, roasted nuts, toasted muesli, crumbled cookies.

Note: You can vary this recipe with the following:
- **Chocolate chia seed pudding:** Add 1 tbsp of cocoa/cacao powder to the basic recipe.
- **Nut/seed butter chia seed pudding:** Add 1 tbsp of nut butter and 2 tbsp of fruit jam to the basic recipe.
- **Blueberry bliss chia seed pudding:** Add ½ cup of blueberries to the basic recipe.
- **Banana split chia seed pudding:** Mash half a banana and add to the basic recipe, and top with whipped cream or vanilla flavoured yoghurt (or dairy-free options).

Dairy-free 'nice' cream

- Low chemical load: contains salicylates, amines
- Free from eggs, lactose, gluten, soy and nuts
- Dairy-free
- FODMAP friendly
- Prep time: 5 minutes
- Overnight for freezing

Ingredients

- 2 cups almond milk (or dairy-free milk of choice)
- ½ cup non-oily nut butter of choice or 1–2 bananas, mashed
- ⅓ cup liquid sweetener of choice (for example, maple syrup, rice bran syrup)
- 1½ tsp vanilla extract

Method

1. Using either a handheld mixer or a high-speed blender, mix all of the ingredients together until smooth.
2. Transfer the mixture into medium-sized square ice cube trays and freeze.
3. Once frozen, blend one to two cubes in a high speed blender until smooth and creamy.
4. Eat straightaway.

Ice cream maker option

1. Add all of the ingredients into an ice cream maker and churn according to manufacturer's instructions.
2. Once the mixture is frozen enough, scoop out and enjoy.
3. Store left over nice cream in an airtight freezer-appropriate container.

Note: You can try the following variations and additions:

- **Mint chocolate chip:** Make sure you use a neutral tasting nut butter, such as cashew or coconut butter in the base recipe. Add ⅛ tsp of pure peppermint extract and chopped chocolate chips to taste. To make it look green, add a little bit of food intolerance friendly food colouring.

- **Chocolate:** Follow the basic recipe above and add ¼ cup of cocoa powder or cacao powder. For a more decadent flavour, add dark chocolate chips and/or pieces of chocolate cake/brownies or muffin.

- **Berry:** Add half a cup of smashed berries and half a cup of diced berries.

- **Raspberry ripe:** Add half a cup of smashed raspberries and a ¼ cup of cocoa or cacao powder.

Basic gluten-free muffin mix

- Low chemical load: contains salicylates, amines
- Free from lactose, gluten, soy and nuts
- Dairy-free
- FODMAP friendly
- Prep time: 5 minutes
- Cooking time: 20 minutes
- Makes 6 large or 12 small muffins

Ingredients

- 1½ cups self-rising flour (gluten-free flour for gluten-free version)
- ½ cup almond flour, or you can use 1/3 cup more of self-rising flour (or gluten-free option)
- 2 tsp gluten-free baking powder/soda
- ½ tsp salt
- 2 large eggs (or equivalent egg replacement)
- ½ cup sugar
- ½ cup vegetable oil
- 1 tbsp lemon juice
- 1 cup whole milk natural yoghurt or lactose-free natural yoghurt or natural coconut yoghurt or other dairy-free options
- 1 tsp vanilla extract

Method

1. Pre-heat oven to 190 °C/375 °F. Line a standard muffin pan with baking paper or baking paper cups.
2. Whisk together all dry ingredients except sugar in a medium bowl and set aside.
3. In another medium bowl or the bowl of a stand mixer fitted with a paddle attachment, add the eggs and sugar, and beat together until light and fluffy – around 5 minutes. A handheld mixer is sufficient if you do not have a stand mixer.
4. Slowly add the oil to the beaten eggs and sugar while the mixer is still running. Then add the lemon juice and continue to mix.

5. Add a third of the flour mixture, followed by around half of the yogurt. Mix this until well combined.

6. Add the remaining yogurt and another third of the flour mixture. Mix until well combined.

7. Add the remaining flour mixture until well combined, scrapping down the sides until the batter is smooth.

8. Stir in only 1 cup in total of your added mix-ins (such as blueberries and chocolate chips) with a rubber spatula and, using an ice-cream scoop or large spoon, add the batter in equal portions to the prepared muffin tin.

9. Bake for around 20 minutes or until muffins are lightly browned or cooked. Inset a toothpick in the centre of the muffin. If it comes out clean, the muffins are cooked.

10. Transfer the muffins to wire rack to cool.

Note: You can mix in the following to the basic mix:

- **White chocolate and raspberry:** ½ cup of each
- **Chocolate chips:** 1 cup
- **Mixed berries:** 1 cup
- **Lemon/orange and poppy seed:** 2 tbsp of poppy seeds and the zest of 1 lemon or orange
- **Apple and cinnamon:** 1 cup of diced apples and 1 tbsp of cinnamon (or to taste)

Basic gluten-free waffles

- Low chemical load: contains salicylates, amines
- Free from lactose, gluten, soy and nuts
- Dairy-free
- FODMAP friendly
- Prep time: 5 minutes
- Cooking time: 5–10 minutes
- Makes 6 waffles

Ingredients

- 2 large eggs (or equivalent egg replacement)
- ¼ cup sugar
- 2 tsp vanilla extract
- ½ cup vegetable oil
- 2 cups plain (all-purpose) flour (or gluten-free flour)
- ½ tsp xanthan gum (leave out if flour already has xanthan gum added or if using wheat flour)
- 4 tsp gluten-free baking powder
- ¼ tsp salt
- 1¾ cups milk or lactose-free/dairy-free milk replacement (almond, cashew, oat milk)

Method

1. Place the eggs (or egg replacement), sugar, vanilla extract and oil in a large bowl and whisk together.
2. Slowly add the flour, xanthan gum (if using), baking powder and salt to the egg mixture, mixing until well combined.
3. Add the milk and stir until batter is smooth and thick.
4. Grease an ice-cream scoop or large spoon and spoon the batter into a pre-heated waffle maker.
5. Cook the waffles as per waffle maker directions or until they are golden brown.
6. Top cooked waffles with lashings of butter, syrup and/or your favourite toppings.

Notes: Cooked waffles can be stored in an air-tight container in the fridge or can be frozen for later. You can reheat the defrosted waffles in a microwave, toaster or sandwich toaster.

Suggested toppings:

- butter and maple syrup
- fresh berries with whipped cream or maple syrup
- chocolate hazelnut spread
- ice cream or sorbet for dairy-free option.

Basic pancake mix

- Low chemical load: contains salicylates, amines
- Free from lactose, gluten, soy and nuts
- Dairy-free
- FODMAP friendly
- Prep time: 5 minutes
- Cooking time: 5–10 minutes
- Makes around 8 pancakes

Ingredients

- 1 large egg (or equivalent egg replacement)
- 2 tbsp sugar (or ¼ cup for a sweeter version)
- 1 tsp vanilla extract
- 2 tbsp vegetable oil
- 1 cup plain (all-purpose) flour (or gluten-free flour)
- ½ tsp xanthan gum (leave out if flour already has xanthan gum added or if using wheat flour)
- 1 tbsp baking powder/soda (or gluten-free equivalent)
- ¼ tsp salt
- ¾ cup whole milk or lactose-free milk or dairy-free alternative (almond, oat, cashew)

Method

1. Whisk together the egg (or egg replacement), sugar, vanilla extract, and vegetable oil in a large bowl.
2. Add the flour, xanthan gum (if using), baking powder/soda and salt to the egg mixture, mixing until well combined.
3. Add the milk and stir until smooth. If you want a thinner pancake batter, stir in an additional 1 to 2 tablespoons of milk or milk alternative.
4. Scoop batter using a ¼ cup measuring cup, and pour into a preheated, non-stick pan.
5. Cook the batter until it starts to bubble on one side and is golden brown on the other. Then flip and leave until the second side is cooked.

6. Repeat instructions 4 and 5 until the remaining batter is cooked.
7. Transfer cooked pancakes onto a plate and serve immediately.

Note: These pancakes can be frozen and reheated in the oven, microwave oven or frypan.

Basic vanilla cookie dough

- Low chemical load: contains salicylates, amines
- Free from lactose, gluten, soy and nuts
- Dairy-free
- FODMAP friendly
- Prep time: 5–10 minutes
- Cooking time: 10 minutes

Ingredients

- 1 cup unsalted butter or dairy-free alternative
- ⅔ cup granulated sugar
- ½ tsp salt
- 1 egg at room temperature
- 1 tsp vanilla extract
- 2 cups plain (all-purpose) flour (or gluten-free flour)

Method

1. Preheat the oven to 180 °C/350 °F.
2. In a large mixing bowl, beat the butter with a handheld mixer until fluffy.
3. Add the sugar and salt to the fluffy butter until well combined.
4. Add the egg and vanilla extract until well combined.
5. Gradually add the flour and beat until well combined. If dough is too thick for the handheld beater, then use a wooden spoon or your hands to mix the flour in.
6. Spoon out the cookie dough in desired amounts onto a parchment paper lined baking sheet and bake for 8–10 minutes or until slightly golden brown.
7. Transfer to a wire rack and cool completely

Note: You can try the following toppings and additions:

- **Unsalted nuts:** Add up to half a cup (or to taste) chopped unsalted nuts of choice. Or place a whole nut in the middle of the uncooked cookie dough mound.

- **Chocolate chips:** Add up to half a cup (or to taste) chocolate chips (milk or dark).
- **Chocolate:** Add quarter of a cup of cacao or cocoa powder to the basic recipe. To avoid the dough getting too dry, you might need to add some extra butter/dairy-free alternative.

Avocado chocolate mouse

- Low to moderate chemical load: contains salicylates, amines and glutamate
- Free from lactose, gluten, soy and nuts
- Dairy-free
- Not suitable for FODMAPs
- Prep time: 5 minutes
- Cooking time: 20 minutes

Ingredients

- 2 large ripe avocados – peeled and pitted
- ¼ cup maple syrup
- ¼ cup cacao/cocoa powder
- 1 ½ tsp vanilla extract
- 1–3 tbsp milk or dairy-free alternative to help bend
- 1½ block dark chocolate, melted

Method

1. Put all ingredients, except the melted chocolate, into a blender and blend until smooth.
2. If you need to add more milk or dairy-free alternative, add it 1 tbsp at a time until you have your desired consistency.
3. Slowly blend the melted chocolate in until mixture is smooth and creamy.
4. Spoon mixture into small cups or ramekins and refrigerate for 2–3 hours.

Note: You can add the following suggested toppings:

- whipped cream or dairy-free alternative
- vanilla yogurt and crumbled cookies or cake
- fresh berries.

Final reflections

WE HAVE COVERED A FAIR bit of ground in this journey through food intolerances and a return to health and wellness. From unravelling the complexities of various food sensitivities to delving into the intricacies of gut health and the microbiome, this journey has been a comprehensive exploration of the relationship between what you eat and how your body responds. The path to wellness involves not only identifying and managing food intolerances, but also embracing a balanced, nutritional lifestyle that contributes to your overall vitality.

Before I sign off, I have summarised the key points of this book that I believe will set you on the right path to managing food intolerances and living a flavourful life.

GET THE RIGHT DIAGNOSIS

I cannot emphasis enough how important it is to get a clinical diagnosis. Trying to guess what you may be intolerant to is like finding a needle in a haystack – virtually impossible.

Here are some tips to finding the right specialists to work with:

- **Contact your local public hospitals to see if they have an allergy unit attached to their services:** Make sure you ask if they diagnose food intolerances as well. This was how I found the allergy unit that helped me.

- **Choose a professional with the right qualifications:** GPs, dietitians, clinical nutritionists, medical specialists or qualified naturopaths are the professionals you should look for.
- **Remember, it is okay to get a second opinion:** If your diagnosis does not seem to fit with your symptoms and you feel the specialist is not listening to what you are saying, then go for it – challenge them. After all, it is your body, and you know it best. You might be a square peg like me and not fit into their textbook round holes.

KNOW WHAT FOOD YOU ARE INTOLERANT TO

Knowing what you are intolerant to is *the key* to managing food intolerances. It allows you to make informed dietary choices and to adopt a lifestyle that aligns with your unique needs. It is imperative to know what you can and can't eat in order to prevent ongoing exposure to food or food groups that are causing a reaction. The solution could be as simple as eliminating gluten or dairy, or as complex as navigating the natural forming chemical maze of salicylates, amines or glutamate.

LOOK OUT FOR PRESERVATIVES AND ADDITIVES

Avoiding preservatives and additives these days is almost impossible. Any food product that comes in a package will have some sort of additive to prolong its shelf life, enhance its colour or flavour, and prevent nasty bacteria from growing and poisoning you. Always check food labels and know which preservatives you need to avoid.

MASTER YOUR SENSITIVITY THRESHOLD

Your sensitivity threshold is the degree to which you can tolerate certain foods and chemicals. This threshold is different for everyone; it depends on how sensitive you are and how much you have eaten.

Once you have a diagnosis and know what food groups, chemicals or preservatives you are sensitive to, learn to work *with* your food intolerance threshold. This is a key factor to managing food intolerances and those nasty symptoms.

GET THOSE DIGESTIVE JUICES FLOWING AND BUILD A HEALTHY GUT MICROBIOME

Embarking on a journey to optimal wellbeing and health involves more than just conscious food choices. Fostering a harmonious relationship with your digestive system includes making a balanced nutritional diet a priority. Practise mindful eating habits, stay hydrated and get in tune to the signals your body is giving. This promotes overall wellbeing and digestive health.

Remember that gut health is very important when it comes to food intolerances. Your gut bacteria have a symbiotic relationship with your body and with your health and wellness. Find the fermented foods that work best with your digestion and food sensitivity and, when experimenting, try not to make moonshine like I did (refer to chapter 3).

REDUCE STRESS, HISTAMINE AND INFLAMMATION LEVELS

Reducing stress, histamine and inflammation levels is essential to managing food intolerances. Stress can cause your digestive system to slow down and malfunction, which makes it the perfect environment for stagnant food particles to ferment and irritate your nervous system. This causes histamine and inflammation levels to rise.

Here are some ways I like to combat stress, helping to reduce histamine and inflammation levels in my sensitive body:

- **Meditation:** I love guided meditations because they spark my imagination and I can visualise the story. This helps me to calm my mind and body and I relax so much that most of the time I fall asleep.
- **Yoga:** Yoga offers myriad benefits that extend beyond physical wellbeing. It is great for your mind and mental health, enhances flexibility, strength and balance, and promotes overall fitness. I find it fascinating how bendy I can be with regular practice.
- **Self-care:** Self-care involves taking steps to prioritise and nurture your own wellbeing. It goes beyond mere indulgence; it is a

commitment to maintaining a healthy and balanced lifestyle.

One of my favourite self-care activities is to take long luxurious bubble baths, where I can immerse myself in the soothing warmth, surrounded by calming fragrance and scented candles. It's a blissful escape from the demands of everyday life and allows me to unwind and relax.

UNDERSTAND HOME FOOD PREPARATION AND COOKING IS KEY

Eating a much higher proportion of home-cooked meals is what I believe will help you to take back nutritional control and conquer food intolerance symptoms. Simple home cooking is returning to the modern kitchen, and people with diets that are limited by food intolerances and digestive disorders will greatly benefit from switching back to home-cooked meals.

FIND PLEASURE IN FOOD AND HAVE FUN WITH FLAVOUR

Food intolerance does not have to be a death sentence for flavour; instead, it can open up a whole new world of creative and delicious alternative choices. It allows you to explore a diverse range of ingredients and innovative cooking techniques to cater to your food intolerance diagnoses without losing out on flavour.

Slap on your own Mad Scientist MasterChef hat and play with your food to create different flavour profiles to suit your dietary needs. Once you do, you are sure to discover some very interesting and tasty flavour blends that you will love to cook over and over again.

DEVELOP A RECIPE LIBRARY

Creating a comprehensive recipe library is a great way to keep variety in meal planning. It's a food lover's death sentence to keep on eating the same things over and over and over again. Don't be afraid to adjust some else's recipe to suit your nutritional needs.

KEEP IN TOUCH!

Travelling the road to health and wellness with other people brings a sense of mutual support, encouragement and shared experiences. This book helps you to understand what food intolerance is, how it affects your body, and how to self-manage symptoms and nutrition. But you may need some extra help – and I'd love to hear from you.

I am in the business of helping people live with their food sensitivities and digestive challenges, without losing out on flavour. I help guide people on their own transformative journey towards gut healing and wellness.

Plus, I have created a community that allows individuals to exchange ideas, their experiences, their motivation, their challenges and triumphs, and support with reaching their health goals. To be part of this community, please visit my website and join the mailing list – where you can also access exclusive recipes, content and program offers. Just go to www.julieannwrightson.com/.

KNOW THIS IS NOT THE END

As my understanding of food intolerance continues to evolve, I believe the way forward involves a multi-faceted approach that is aimed at improving diagnosis, management and overall wellbeing for people with food intolerances. I am really excited to get my hands on any ongoing research into gut health and the microbiome, because it promises to help unravel fascinating connections between our digestive system, food intolerances and overall health. Exploring the latest findings in this field not only fuels my curiosity but also holds potential to enhance my understanding of how the microbiome influences various aspects of health.

Before I go, here is my final message to you: *Knowledge is power.* Let that sink in for a bit.

When I set out on my own food intolerant lifestyle, I knew nothing about it other than what to eat and what not to eat. I discovered that the more I knew about what was happening to my body, what food made me sick and how to manage my diet, the more quickly I returned to a balanced state of health. Identifying and addressing your food intolerances allows you to make informed choices, promotes digestive comfort, enhances your energy levels and supports your overall health. Being mindful of the food you are intolerant to empowers you to take back control and to live a healthy, flavourful life. I wish you the best of luck.

Appendices

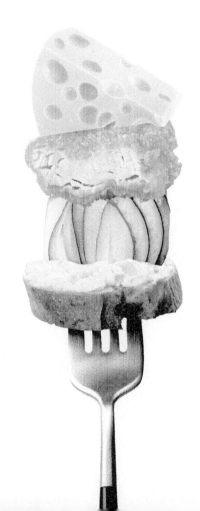

APPENDIX A

Levels of salicylates, amines, glutamates in various food types

Scale: LM = Low to moderate H = High VH = Very high

Fruit	Salicylates	Amines	Glutamate
Apple:			
all varieties	LM		
dried	LM		
Apricot:			
fresh	LM		
dried			VH
Avocado:			
just ripe	H	H	
soft & mashable		VH	VH
Banana:			
just ripe		LM	
ripe		H	
dried		VH	
Berries:			
blackberry	VH	VH	
blackcurrant	VH	VH	
blueberry	H		
boysenberry	VH	VH	
cranberry	VH	VH	
mulberry	H		
raspberry	VH	VH	
redcurrant	VH	VH	
strawberry	VH		
Cherry	VH	VH	

Fruit	Salicylates	Amines	Glutamate
Citrus fruits:			
grapefruit	VH	VH	
lemon	VH	VH	
lime	VH	VH	
mandarin	VH	VH	
orange	VH	VH	
tangelo	VH	VH	
Coconut:			
fresh	VH	VH	
dried	H	H	
Custard apple	LM	H	
Dates:			
fresh	VH	VH	
dried	VH	VH	
Dragon fruit	H		
Dried fruits:			
currants	VH		
prunes	VH	VH	VH
raisins	VH	VH	VH
sultanas	VH	VH	VH
Figs:			
fresh	H	H	
dried	VH	VH	
Fruit confectionary:			
cordials	VH	VH	VH
drinks	VH	VH	VH
jams	VH	VH	VH
jellies	VH	VH	VH
juices	VH	VH	VH
Grapes: green & red	VH	VH	VH
Guava		H	
Kiwifruit		VH	VH
Lychee	H		
Mango:			
fresh	H	H	
dried			VH

Fruit	Salicylates	Amines	Glutamate

Melon:
  rockmelon
  honeydew
  watermelon
	H	LM
		H	

Nectarine	H		

Papaya/pawpaw:
  fresh
  dried
		H	VH

Peach	H		
Pear	LM		
Pineapple			VH
Plum	VH	VH	VH
Pomegranate	H	LM	
Rhubarb	H	LM	
Starfruit	H	LM	
Tamarillo	H	H	

Tomato:
  fresh, peeled & sliced
  dried, sun-dried, juice
  puree, paste & sauce
	H
	VH
	VH
		H
		VH
		VH
			H
			VH
			VH

Vegetables	Salicylates	Amines	Glutamate
Alfalfa	H		
Artichoke	H		
Asparagus	LM		
Bamboo shoots: tinned & fresh	LM		

Beans:
  butter, French, string, snake
  bean shoots
  broad beans, fava beans
  mung bean sprouts
	LM
	LM
	VH
	LM
		VH	

Beetroot: tinned & fresh	LM		
Bok choy	LM		
Broccoli/broccolini	H	H	H

Vegetables	Salicylates	Amines	Glutamate
Brussel sprouts	LM		
Cabbage: red, green, savoy, wombok	LM		
Capsicum: green, red, yellow, orange	VH		
Carrots	LM		
Cauliflower	H	H	
Celery	LM		
Chicory	VH		
Choko	LM		
Corn	H		H
Cucumbers	LM		
Eggplant	VH	VH	
Endive	H		
Fennel	H		
Herbs & spices (dried & fresh):			
basil	VH		
chilli	LM		
chives	LM		
garlic	VH		
ginger	VH		
mint	VH		
turmeric	VH		
curry mixes	VH		
parsley	LM		
saffron threads	LM		
Leek	LM		
Lettuce:			
iceberg, cos, red & green	LM		
coral, red & green oak	LM		
Mushrooms & truffles	VH	VH	VH
Olives	VH	VH	
Onions:			
red, yellow	VH		
spring onions	H		
shallots	LM		

Vegetables	Salicylates	Amines	Glutamate

Peas:
    green, snow, sugar snap
    snow pea sprouts
	LM
	H		

Pickled vegetables: cucumbers, gherkins, olives, onions	VH	VH	VH
Potato: all varieties	LM		
Pumpkin: all varieties	LM		
Radish	H		
Rocket	H	H	
Seaweed (Nori)	VH	VH	VH
Spinach: English, silverbeet, Chinese	VH	VH	VH
Swede	LM		
Sweet potato/kumara	LM		
Turnip	LM		
Vegetable juices, soups, & stocks: commercial cubes, liquid & powder	VH	VH	VH
Water chestnut	H		
Watercress	H		
Zucchini	LM		

Meat	Salicylates	Amines	Glutamate

Beef:
    fresh, not aged
    aged
		LM
		VH
			LM
			VH

Chicken:
    fresh
    chicken skin
		LM
		H	

Deli meats:
    beef – corned, dried, jerky
    salami, smoked, seasoned
    chicken – pressed
    nuggets, seasoned, smoked
    devon
    ham
    bacon
	VH
	VH
	VH
	VH
	VH
		VH
		VH
		VH
		VH
		VH
		VH
		VH
			VH
			VH
			VH
			VH
			VH

Meat	Salicylates	Amines	Glutamate
Duck		LM	
Game meat: venison, kangaroo, emu		H	
Lamb		LM	
Meat pastes	VH	VH	VH
Meat pies	VH	VH	VH
Offal: liver, kidneys, brains, tripe	VH	VH	VH
Pork		H	
Rabbit		LM	
Sausages	VH	VH	VH
Turkey		H	
Veal		LM	

Seafood	Salicylates	Amines	Glutamate

Canned or bottled:
  tuna
  salmon
  anchovies
  oysters
  muscles
  pilchards
		VH
		VH
		VH
		VH
		VH
		VH	

Fish:
  dried, pickled, salted, smoked
  fish roe – caviar
  pastes, sauces, and marinades
  fish fingers
  fish – frozen
	
	VH
		VH
		VH
		VH
		H
		H
			
			VH

Seafood – fresh:
  white fish
  salmon
  tuna
  crab
  lobster
  calamari
  sea scallops
  natural oysters
  muscles
		LM
		LM
		LM
		LM
		LM
		LM
		LM
		LM
		LM	

Surimi: fake crab meat		VH	

Legumes	Salicylates	Amines	Glutamate
Bean mixes:			
three, four & five	LM	LM	
mixed beans with sauce	VH	VH	
baked beans in sauce	VH	VH	VH
Black eye beans	LM	LM	
Borlotti beans	LM	LM	
Broad beans	VH	VH	
Butter beans	LM	LM	
Cannellini beans	LM	LM	
Chickpeas:			
dried, canned	LM	LM	
felafel	VH	VH	
hummus	VH	VH	
Haricot beans	LM	LM	
Lentils	LM	LM	
Lima beans	LM	LM	
Lupin	LM	LM	
Mung bean	LM	LM	
Red kidney beans	LM	LM	
Soup mixes: dried	LM	LM	
Soya beans	LM	LM	
Split peas	LM	LM	
White beans	LM	LM	

Nuts & seeds	Salicylates	Amines	Glutamate
Nuts – raw:			
almond	H	H	
Brazil	H	H	
cashew	LM	LM	
chestnut	H	H	
hazelnut	H	H	
macadamia	H	H	
peanut	H	H	
pecan	H	H	
pinenut	H	H	
pistachio	H	H	
walnut	H	H	

Nuts & seeds	Salicylates	Amines	Glutamate
All nut meal	VH	VH	
Nut pastes: peanut butter; all other nut pastes	VH	VH	
All roasted nuts	VH	VH	
Seeds – raw:			
black nigella	VH	VH	
linseed	H	H	
mustard	VH	VH	
poppy	LM	LM	
pumpkin/pepitas	H	H	
sesame	H	H	
sunflower	H	H	
Seed pastes: tahini, all other seed pastes	VH	VH	

Dairy, lactose free & dairy alternatives	Salicylates	Amines	Glutamate
Dairy:			
butter, ghee, margarine		LM	
cheese: mild, cheddar tasty		H	
cheese: feta, haloumi		H	
cheese: brie, camembert, parmesan		VH	VH
cheese: flavoured, fruit	VH	VH	VH
cream, sour cream		LM	
milk: plain		LM	
milk: flavoured with chocolate, banana, strawberry	VH	VH	VH
yoghurt: natural, Greek, plain, vanilla flavoured	VH	LM	
yoghurt: with fruit flavours		VH	VH
Lactose free:			
dairy free margarine, Nuttelex		LM	
cheese: mild, cheddar tasty		H	
cheese: feta, haloumi		H	
cheese: brie, camembert, parmesan		VH	VH
cheese: flavoured, fruit	VH	VH	VH
cream, sour cream		LM	
milk		LM	
milk: flavoured with chocolate, banana, strawberry	VH	VH	VH
yoghurt: natural, Greek, plain, vanilla flavoured		LM	
yoghurt: with fruit flavours	VH	VH	VH

Dairy, lactose free & dairy alternatives	Salicylates	Amines	Glutamate
Dairy alternatives:			
nut cheeses with nutritional yeast & fruits	VH	VH	VH
nut cheeses without nutritional yeast	H	H	
nut cheese: cashew	LM	LM	
nut milk: almond, macadamia	H	H	
nut milk: cashew	LM	LM	
yoghurt: coconut without flavouring	H	H	
yoghurt: coconut with fruit flavouring	VH	VH	VH
Soy:			
soy cream cheese		LM	
soy hard cheese		H	
soy custard		LM	
soy drinks: milk, vanilla, carob		LM	
soy yoghurt: plain, vanilla		LM	
tofu: firm		LM	
tofu: soft		LM	

Gluten-free products	Salicylates	Amines	Glutamate
Breads:			
homemade or commercial using low-chemical gluten-free grains, flour mixes without maize flour	LM	LM	
breads containing dried fruit, nuts, coconut, vinegar, propionates (preservative 280–283)	VH	VH	VH
corn bread	H		H
sourdough	LM	LM	
Baked goods:			
biscuits, cakes, muesli bars, pastries containing fresh coconut, maize flour	H	H	H
biscuits, cakes, muesli bars, pastries containing chocolate, coconut fruit, nuts, jam, spices, antioxidants (310–312, 319–321) colours, preservatives	VH	VH	VH

Gluten-free products	Salicylates	Amines	Glutamate
Baked goods – homemade or commercial using low-chemical gluten-free grains. flour mixes without maize flours:			
biscuits	LM	LM	
cakes	LM	LM	
crumpets	LM	LM	
muffins	LM	LM	
pancakes	LM	LM	
pappadums	LM	LM	
pikelets	LM	LM	
pizza bases	LM	LM	
pretzels	LM	LM	
rice paper	LM	LM	
scones	LM	LM	
shortbread	LM	LM	
Grains & flours:			
amaranth: flour, flakes, puffed, grain	LM		
arrowroot flour	LM		
besan (chickpea) flour	LM		
buckwheat flour, grain, cereal	LM		
corn: cornmeal	H		H
maize cornflour cornstarch	H		H
millet, flour, meal, flakes, puffed	LM		
polenta	H		H
potato flour	LM		
psyllium husks, powder	LM		
quinoa, flour, flakes, puffed, grains	LM		
rice: white, brown, basmati, jasmine, wild, rice bran, rice crumbs, rice flour, rice flakes, puffed rice, ground rice	LM		
sago	LM		
sorghum flour	LM		
tapioca starch	LM		
Pasta & noodles:			
buckwheat	LM		
chickpea	LM		
legume	LM		
maze, corn pasta	H		
noodles, coloured, flavoured	VH	VH	VH
quinoa	LM		
rice	LM		

Gluten-free products	Salicylates	Amines	Glutamate
Snack foods:			
flavoured, containing fruit, honey, nuts, cheese, herbs, soy sauce, spices tamari, antioxidants (310–312, 319–321) colours, flavours (620–635) including potato chips, flavoured corn chips, flavoured rice crackers	VH	VH	VH
Rice cakes & corn thins containing corns, sesame, sunflower	H	H	H
Unflavoured corn chips, tacos, rice cakes	VH	VH	

Pantry items	Salicylates	Amines	Glutamate
Baking aids:			
agar agar	LM	LM	
baking powder	LM	LM	
bicarbonate soda	LM		
cornstarch, corn flour, maize flour	LM		LM
cream of tartar	LM	LM	
gelatine: leaf & powder		LM	
gums: guar, xanthan	LM	LM	
lecithin		LM	
vanilla: pods, natural essence	LM	LM	LM
Colours:			
artificial	VH	VH	VH
natural concentrate	H	H	H

Pantry items	Salicylates	Amines	Glutamate
Confectionary:			
cacao powder		VH	
caramels	LM		
carob	LM		
chewing gum	VH		
chocolate: dark & milk		VH	
chocolate: white		H	
cocoa powder		VH	
crystallised ginger	VH		
honeycomb	LM		
liquorice	VH		
marshmallows	LM		
meringues	LM		
sweets: coloured	VH	VH	
sweets: fruit	VH	VH	
sweets: mint	VH		
sweets: peppermint	VH		
toffee	LM		
Turkish delight	VH		
Dressings:			
mayonnaise: all commercial	VH	VH	
mayonnaise: homemade with LM oil	LM	LM	
tahini	VH	VH	
salad dressings: all commercial	VH	VH	VH
Fats:			
copha	H	H	
suet		H	
lard		LM	
Fermented: all products	VH	VH	VH
Flavouring:			
curry powder	VH	VH	
enhancers: HVP & TVP	VH	VH	VH
essences	VH	VH	VH
flavouring powders, mixes, syrups	VH	VH	VH
food colours: artificial	VH	VH	VH
food colours: natural	H	H	H
meat extracts	VH	VH	VH
mustards	VH	VH	VH
tandoori powder mix	VH	VH	VH
Herbs & spices: all dried & fresh	VH	VH	VH

Pantry items	Salicylates	Amines	Glutamate
Oils:			
almond oil	VH	VH	
avocado oil	VH	VH	
canola oil	LM	LM	
coconut oil	H	H	
corn oil	LM		
cottonseed oil	LM		
flavoured, infused oils	VH	VH	
grape seed oil	VH	VH	
linseed oil	VH		
mustard seed oil	VH	VH	
olive oil: extra virgin, cold pressed	VH	VH	
olive oil: pure, classic, traditional	H	H	
olive oil: extra light, light, mild, mellow	LM	LM	
peanut oil	H	H	
rice bran oil	LM	LM	
safflower oil	LM	LM	
sesame oil	VH	VH	
sunflower oil	LM	LM	
vegetable oil	H		
walnut oil	VH	VH	
Pastes:			
curry	VH	VH	
fish	VH	VH	VH
fruit	VH		
horseradish	VH		
meat		VH	VH
miso		VH	VH
pâtés	VH	VH	VH
pesto	VH		
tamarind	VH	VH	VH
tomato: paste & puree	VH	VH	VH
wasabi	VH		
Salts:			
chicken	VH	VH	VH
flavoured	VH	VH	VH
iodised	LM		
rock	LM		
sea	LM		
table	LM		

Pantry items	Salicylates	Amines	Glutamate
Sauces:			
all commercial	VH	VH	VH
BBQ	VH	VH	VH
fish		VH	VH
gravy: commercial	VH	VH	VH
gravy: homemade with meat juice		H	H
miso		VH	VH
mustard	VH	VH	VH
oyster		VH	VH
sriracha	VH	VH	VH
soy		VH	VH
tabasco		VH	VH
tamari		VH	VH
tempeh		VH	VH
teriyaki		VH	VH
tomato, ketchup	VH	VH	VH
Worcestershire	VH	VH	VH
Spreads:			
capers	VH		
chutney	VH	VH	VH
fruit, jams	VH	VH	VH
mustard	VH	VH	VH
pickles	VH	VH	VH
relishes	VH	VH	VH
yeast: Vegemite, Marmite, Promite	VH	VH	VH
Stock:			
bone broth: commercial	VH	VH	VH
liquid: commercial	VH	VH	VH
liquid: homemade	LM	LM	LM
powders, cubes: commercial	VH	VH	VH
Sweet spreads:			
chocolate		VH	
chocolate hazelnut		VH	
fruit butter	VH	VH	
fruit conserve	VH	VH	VH
fruit jam	VH	VH	VH
fruit jelly	VH	VH	VH
fruit preserves	VH	VH	VH
marmalade	VH	VH	
nut spreads	VH	VH	

Pantry items	Salicylates	Amines	Glutamate
Sugar:			
brown sugar	LM		
caster sugar	LM		
coconut sugar	LM	LM	
icing sugar	LM		
jaggery	H		
liquid glucose	LM		
malt		LM	
palm sugar	LM	LM	
raw sugar	H		
white sugar	LM		
Syrups:			
caramel syrup		LM	
chocolate syrup		VH	
coconut syrup	H	H	
fruit syrups	VH		
golden syrup	LM		
honey	VH		
maple syrup: pure & flavoured	LM		
molasses	VH		
rice syrup	LM		
treacle	VH		
Vinegar:			
apple cider	VH	VH	
balsamic	VH	VH	VH
malt		LM	
red wine	VH	VH	
rice wine		VH	
white wine	VH	VH	
Yeast:			
bakers: fresh, dried	LM	LM	LM
brewer's	H	H	H
extracts	VH	VH	VH
flakes	VH	VH	VH
nutritional seasonings	VH	VH	VH

Drinks & alcohol	Salicylates	Amines	Glutamate
Alcohol:			
beer: all	VH	VH	
flavoured spirits and ciders: all	H	H	
liqueurs: all	VH	VH	VH
spirits: bourbon, brandy, cognac,	VH	VH	VH
pre-mixes, port, rum, sherry			
spirits: gin, vodka, whisky	LM	LM	LM
wine: champagne, sparkling	VH	VH	
wine: red, white, rosé	VH	VH	VH
Coffee:			
all	H		
coffee substitutes	LM		
Fruit flavoured drinks:			
syrups, cordials, fruit mixes, tomato juice	VH	VH	VH
fruit juice: all	VH	VH	VH
fruit juice: pear	LM		
Soft drinks/sodas:			
all	VH	VH	
flavoured mineral water	VH	VH	VH
ginger beer	VH	VH	
cola drinks	VH	VH	
lemonade	LM		
tonic water	LM		
Tea:			
black tea	VH		
fruit & herbal teas	VH		
Chai spiced tea	VH	VH	
camomile tea	H		
iced tea mixes	VH	VH	
Vegetable juice: all	VH	VH	VH
Water: fruit flavoured	VH	VH	

APPENDIX B

Foods with low FODMAP levels

Vegetables

- Alfalfa
- Bamboo shoots
- Bean sprouts
- Beetroot – cooked, canned and/or pickled
- Bitter melon (karela)
- Bok choy
- Broccoli – whole
- Brussel sprouts
- Cabbage – green & red
- Capsicum (bell peppers) – red, green, yellow, orange
- Carrots
- Celery & celery root (celeriac)
- Collard greens
- Corn – fresh, canned
- Cucumber
- Edamame
- Eggplant (aubergine)
- Fennel
- Green beans
- Kale
- Leek – green leaves only
- Lettuce – all types
- Okra
- Olives – green and black
- Onions (green tops) – the green tops of scallions or green onions only
- Parsnip
- Peas – green and snow
- Potato – all varieties
- Pumpkin – all varieties
- Radish – daikon
- Rocket (arugula)
- Seaweed (nori)
- Silverbeet (chard)
- Spinach – baby, English, Chinese, water
- Squash (summer & spaghetti)
- Swede (rutabaga)
- Sweet potato
- Swiss chard
- Tomato – all varieties, tomatillo
- Turnip
- Water chestnuts
- Yam
- Zucchini (courgette or marrow)

Herbs & spices

- Garlic (dried and fresh) and powdered onion are NOT FODMAP friendly.
- All other herbs and spices are FODMAP friendly.

Fruit

- Banana – unripe
- Berries – blueberries (bilberries), cranberries (lingonberries), raspberry, strawberry
- Coconut – cream, flesh, water
- Dragon fruit
- Grapes – all varieties
- Guava – ripe
- Jack fruit (bread fruit)
- Kiwi fruit
- Lemon
- Lime
- Mandarin (clementine)
- Melon – cantaloupe (rockmelon), honeydew
- Orange
- Papaya
- Passionfruit
- Pawpaw
- Pineapple
- Rhubarb
- Star fruit (carambola)
- Tamarind
- Tangelo

Legumes

Legumes consist of a class of carbohydrates called oligosaccharides that can be difficult to digest. The following legumes can be consumed on a low FODMAP diet; however, it will depend on what an individual can tolerate.

Generally, 20–40 grams is tolerated by most people. Make sure the beans have been soaked for at least 24 hours and are cooked. If eating canned beans, thoroughly rinse off the liquid the beans have been soaking in.

- Adzuki beans
- Black beans
- Butter beans (lima beans)
- Chickpeas (garbanzo beans) – canned, dried
- Lentils – in small amounts
- Moth beans
- Mung beans – green, cooked

Nuts & seeds

- Almonds
- Brazil nuts
- Chestnuts
- Chia seeds
- Dill seeds
- Flax seeds
- Hazelnuts
- Hemp seeds
- Linseeds

Meat, seafood & animal products

- Beef – plain, ground
- Game meats – venison, bison, kangaroo
- Lamb – plain, ground
- Pork – plain, ground
- Poultry – chicken, turkey, duck
- Processed meats – deli meat, corned meat, bacon, prosciutto, chorizo without high FODMAP ingredients.
- Seafood – fresh, canned fish, lobster, prawns (shrimp), crab, muscles, oysters, clams, squid (calamari)
- Eggs – all

Dairy & substitutes

Most people believe that they cannot have dairy products on a low FODMAP diet. This is because regular dairy products do contain the sugar lactose, which is also a type of FODMAP. Small amounts of lactose generally are not an issue on a low FODMAP diet; however, if you are lactose intolerant you will need to avoid diary completely.

- Cheese – brie, camembert, cheddar, cottage, cream cheese, feta, goat cheese, haloumi, mozzarella, paneer, parmesan, ricotta, Swiss
- Cream – lactose-free, non-dairy alternatives
- Ghee (clarified butter)
- Ice cream & sorbets – dairy-free alternatives such as coconut ice cream and FODMAP friendly fruit sorbets.
- Margarine (Nuttelex for dairy-free alternative)
- Milk – almond milk, hemp milk, lactose-free milk, macadamia milk, oat milk, rice milk
- Tofu – all varieties
- Yoghurt – lactose-free, coconut, Greek or goat milk yoghurt

Flours & grains

- Buckwheat – whole, flour, noodles
- Corn flour (maize flour) – tortillas
- Millet – grain flour
- Oats – oat-based products
- Pasta – wheat based and gluten free
- Polenta
- Potato flour
- Quinoa – grain, flour
- Rice – white, brown, flour, noodles, basmati, rice bran, rice flakes
- Sorghum flour
- Starches – arrowroot, psyllium, maize, potato, & tapioca
- Teff flour
- Wheat – bulgar

Sweeteners

- Artificial – aspartame, acesulfame K, erythritol (E968/968), stevia, Splenda saccharin
- Glucose
- Golden syrup
- Jaggery
- Maple syrup
- Rice malt syrup
- Sucrose
- Sugar – brown, white, raw

Condiments

- Acia powder
- Baking powder/soda
- Cacao – powder
- Capers – in vinegar, salted
- Cocoa – powder
- Gelatine
- Jams (jelly) – strawberry, raspberry, marmalade
- Mayonnaise
- Miso paste
- Mustard – all
- Nut butters – almond, peanut
- Nutritional yeast
- Pesto – commercial jar
- Salt & pepper
- Sauce – barbecue, fish sauce, tomato (ketchup), oyster, soy, sriracha (hot chilli), sweet & sour sauce,
- Shrimp (prawn) paste
- Tahini paste
- Tamarind paste
- Vanilla essence
- Vegemite (Marmite)
- Vinegars – apple cider, balsamic, rice wine, malt
- Wasabi – powder, paste

Fats & oils

- Butter – ghee (clarified butter)
- Lard
- Oils – avocado, canola, coconut, olive, peanut, rice bran, sesame, sunflower, vegetable

Beverages & alcohol

- Alcohol – beer, clear spirits (vodka, gin), whiskey, wine (red, white & sparkling).
- Coconut – water, milk
- Coffee – black, regular, decaffeinated, instant
- Fizzy drinks (soft drinks, soda) – sugar free, diet, lemonade, cola
- Fruit juices – low FODMAP fruits only.
- Tea – black, Chia, fruit teas, peppermint, green, white, herbal

APPENDIX C

Artificial and nutritive sweeteners approved for use

Artificial sweeteners approved for consumption by FSANZ

Name	Description
Acesulphame K (950) Hermestas Gold® Sunnett®	Found in soft drinks, protein shakes, drink mixes, frozen desserts, baked goods, candy, chewing gums and as a tabletop sweetener. Acesulphame K is 200 times sweeter than sugar. Its naturally bitter aftertaste is masked by adding other sweeteners such as sucralose or aspartame.
Alitame (956) Aclame®	Used in a range of foods that include bakery goods, water-based flavoured drinks, dairy-based drinks and desserts, cream, edible ices, jams, confectionary and dietary foods. Alitame is 2000 times sweeter than sugar and can be used in 'tabletop' sweeteners (provided in cafes and airports, for example).
Aspartame (951) Equal®, Equal Spoonful® Hermesetas Gold® NutraSweet®	Used in many different diet products to sweeten food without the calories. It is used in a wide variety of diet foods such as drinks, dairy products, confectionary, frozen desserts, powdered baking products, cereals and preserves.
Cyclamate (952) Sucaryl®	Has a wide range of applications and can be combined with other artificial sweeteners. Found in tabletop sweeteners in tablet, powder and liquid form, instant beverages, soft drinks, shakes, iced teas, sports drinks, breakfast cereals, dairy products, cakes and baked goods, fruit preserves and jams, biscuits, chocolate, salad dressings, toothpaste and mouthwash.

Name	Description
Neotame (961)	A food additive that is 13,000 times sweeter than table sugar and is approved for use in a wide variety of food products, such as soft drinks, baked goods, dairy products and confectionary. Neotame can be combined with other sweeteners, and is also used as a flavour enhancer (E961).
Saccharin (954) Hermesetas® Sugarella® Sugarine® Sweetex®	The oldest artificial sweetener, first discovered around 1879 by chemists Ira Remsen and Constantin Fahlberg. Saccharin is between 200 and 700 times sweeter than sugar and is usually paired with another sweetener to help soften its bitter aftertaste. Saccharin is approved by FSANZ for use in soft drinks, baked goods, confectionary and juices. It can also be used as a table-top sugar (Sugarine).
Sucralose (955) Splenda®	Derived from sucrose and around 650 times sweeter than sugar. It has no bitter aftertaste and is used in a broad range of food and beverages, including soft drinks, bread, cereals, baked goods, confectionary and salad dressings, and as a table-top sugar.

Nutritive sweeteners approved for consumption by FSANZ

Name	Description
Fructose (no code)	Also known as fruit sugar, with the same kilojoules as sugar but much sweeter. Fructose is found in fruits, carbonated beverages, cereals, cereal bars, juices, confectionary, baked goods, honey and desserts. Concentrated levels of fructose can be found in high-fructose corn syrup, agave nectar, crystalline fructose, sorbitol, corn syrup solids and sugar alcohols.
Isomalt (953)	A combination of two sugar alcohols: mannitol (967) and sorbitol (420). Isomalt is used as a sweetener, bulking, anti-caking and glazing agent in low-calorie confectionary, chewing gum, chocolates, ice creams, baked goods, ready-to-eat cereals, fruit preserves, smoked fish and meats, infant formulas, cough syrups, vitamin and mineral supplements, pan-coated tablets and lozenges.

Name	Description
Sugar alcohols	Lactitol (966): a processed sugar alcohol (not the same alcohol as the fun stuff) approved by FANZS to use in food; however, mostly used to relieve adult constipation. Lactitol tends to aggravate people with food intolerances. Mannitol (421): used as the dust that *coats* chewing gum and stops it from absorbing moisture. Mannitol is TGA (Therapeutic Goods of Australia) approved and is used in pharmaceuticals such as Bronchitol (a powder used in nebulisers for the treatment of lung conditions). Maltitol (967), Xylitol (965), Sorbitol (420): all processed sugar alcohols. They are not quite as sweet as sugar and have half the calories. They are used in baked goods, confectionary, ready-made desserts, dairy – and pretty much any sweet item you can think of.
Maltodextrin (no code)	A common additive made from corn, rice, potato starch or wheat. It is a highly processed white powder often used as a thickener or filler in processed foods, including instant puddings, gelatines, sauces and salad dressings. It can be combined with other intense sweeteners and is used as a thickener in personal care items such as skin lotion and hair products.
Polydextrose (1200)	A low-calorie carbohydrate made by combining D-glucose and sorbitol derived from cornstarch and citric acid. Mostly used as a thickener and stabiliser in non-sweet baked goods, dairy products, ice creams, breakfast cereals, fruit spreads, chicken nuggets, burgers, chewing gum, infant formulas and as a fat or sugar replacement in low-calorie foods.
Thaumatin (957)	A low-calorie protein-based sweetener and flavour enhancer. Used for its flavour-enhancing abilities (E957), not as a sweetener, due to its liquorice-like aftertaste.

APPENDIX D

List of food preservatives and additives code numbers

Flavour enhancers	
Glutamate – MSG	620–625
Disodium guanylate	627
Disodium inosinate	631
Combined 627 & 631	635
Hydrolysed vegetable protein – HVP	
Textured vegetable protein – TVP	
Preservatives	
Sorbates	200–203
Benzoates	210–218
Sulphites	220–228
Nitrates/nitrites	249–252
Propionates	280–283
Antioxidants	310–312, 319–321
Mineral salts	450, 451, 452
Colours	
Artificial colours	102, 104, 110, 122, 123, 124, 127, 129, 132, 133, 142, 143, 151, 155
Natural colour	160b

Endnotes

1   Manzel, A, Muller, DN, Hafler, DA et al (2014), 'Role of "Western diet" in inflammatory autoimmune diseases', Curr Allergy Asthma Rep 14, 404, https://doi.org/10.1007/s11882-013-0404-6.

2   For more on ultra-processed foods, see Anne-Marie Stelluti (2019), 'Everything in moderation? Focusing on ultra-processed foods', GI Society, Canadian Society of Intestinal Research.

3   Thangam EB, Jemima EA, Singh H, Baig MS, Khan M, Mathias CB, Church MK, Saluja R (2018), 'The role of histamine and histamine receptors in mast cell-mediated allergy and inflammation: The hunt for new therapeutic targets', Front Immunol, Aug 13;9:1873. doi: 10.3389/fimmu.2018.01873. PMID: 30150993; PMCID: PMC6099187; Caffarelli C, Di Mauro D, Mastrorilli C, Bottau P, Cipriani F, Ricci G (2018), 'Solid food introduction and the development of food allergies', Nutrients, Nov 17;10(11):1790. doi: 10.3390/nu10111790. PMID: 30453619; PMCID: PMC6266759.

4   Clarke, L, McQueen, J, Samild, A, Swain, A (1996), 'The dietary management of food allergy and food intolerance in children and adults', Dietitians Association of Australia review paper, *Australian Journal of Nutrition and Dietetics*, 53:3.

5   Skypala IJ, Williams M, Reeves L, Meyer R, Venter C (2015), 'Sensitivity to food additives, vaso-active amines and salicylates: a review of the evidence', *Clin Transl Allergy*, Oct 13;5:34. doi: 10.1186/s13601-015-0078-3. PMID: 26468368; PMCID: PMC4604636; Lacy BE, Chey WD, Lembo AJ (2015), 'New and emerging treatment options for irritable bowel syndrome', *Gastroenterol Hepatol* (N Y), Apr;11(4 Suppl 2):1-19. PMID: 26491416; PMCID: PMC4612133.

6   Tuck, CJ, Biesiekierski, JR, Schmid-Grendelmeier, P, Pohl, D (2019), 'Food intolerances', *Nutrients*, Jul 22;11(7):1684.

7   Alcock, J, Maley, CC, Aktipis, CA (2014), 'Is eating behavior manipulated by the gastrointestinal microbiota? Evolutionary pressures and potential mechanisms', *Bioessays*, Oct;36(10):940–9.

8   Tomova, A, Bukovsky, I, Rembert, E, Yonas, W, Alwarith, J, Barnard, ND, Kahleova, H (2019), 'The effects of vegetarian and vegan diets on gut microbiota', *Front Nutr*, Apr 17;6:47.

9   Konturek, PC, Brzozowski, T, Konturek, SJ (2011), 'Stress and the gut: Pathophysiology, clinical consequences, diagnostic approach and treatment options', *J Physiol Pharmacol*, Dec;62(6):591–9.

10 Peuhkuri, K, Vapaatalo, H, Korpela, R (2010), 'Even low-grade inflammation impacts on small intestinal function', *World J Gastroenterol*, Mar 7;16(9):1057–62.

11 Liu, J, Liu, Y, Li, X (2023), 'Effects of intestinal flora on polycystic ovary syndrome', *Front Endocrinol* (Lausanne), Mar 9;14:1151723.

12 Swain, AR (1998), 'The role of natural salicylates in food intolerance', PhD thesis, The University of Sydney.

13 Skypala, IJ, Williams, M, Reeves, L, Meyer, R, Venter, C (2015), 'Sensitivity to food additives, vaso-active amines and salicylates: A review of the evidence', *Clin Transl Allergy*, Oct 13;5:34.

14 Premont, RT, Gainetdinov, RR, Caron, MG (2001), 'Following the trace of elusive amines', *Proc Natl Acad Sci USA*, Aug 14;98(17):9474–5.

15 David, TJ (2000), 'Adverse reactions and intolerance to foods', *British Medical Bulletin*, 56(1):34–50.

16 Hrubisko, M, Danis, R, Huorka, M, Wawruch, M (2021), 'Histamine intolerance – the more we know the less we know. A review', *Nutrients*, 13(7):2228,

17 (2010), 'PEA – a natural antidepressant', Clinical Education, https://www.clinicaleducation.org/resources/reviews/pea-a-natural-antidepressant/.

18 Loï, C, Cynober, L (2022), 'Glutamate: A safe nutrient, not just a simple additive', *Ann Nutr Metab*, 78(3):133–146.

19 WebMD Editorial Contributors (2023), 'What to know about nightshade vegetables', WebMD.

20 Myhill, S (updated 2022), 'Fermentation in the gut and CFS', https://www. DoctorMyhill.co.uk, https://www.drmyhill.co.uk/wiki/Fermentation_in_the_gut_and_CFS.

21 Davis, W (2015), 'Loading up on galacto-oligosaccharides', Dr. Davis Infinite Health, https://drdavisinfinitehealth.com/2015/09/loading-up-on-galacto-oligosaccharides/.

22 Ipatenco, S (2018), 'Good food sources for disaccharides', *Week&*, 27 December.

23 'Monosaccharides or simple sugars', NutrientsReview.com, https://www.nutrientsreview.com/carbs/monosaccharides-simple-sugars.html.

24 Scott, A (2020) 'What are polyols?', A Little Bit Yummy, https://alittlebityummy.com/blog/what-are-polyols/.

25 'FODMAPs and irritable bowel syndrome', Monash University, https://www.monashfodmap.com/about-fodmap-and-ibs/.

26 'Dessert recipes', Medieval Recipes, https://www.medieval-recipes.com/recipes/desserts/.

27 'What is sugar', AB Sugar, https://makingsenseofsugar.com/all-about-sugar/what-is-sugar/.

28 (2007), 'Sugar intolerance', Eating for Energy, https://www.eatingforenergy. com/sugar-intolerance/.

29 'Lactose intolerance', MedlinePlus, National Library of Medicine, https:// medlineplus.gov/genetics/condition/lactose-intolerance/#frequency.

30 'Dairy intolerance: Lactose intolerance, casein allergy', Food Intolerance Institute, https://www.foodintol.com/dairy-intolerance.

31 Thomson, H (2014), 'Artificial sweeteners linked to glucose intolerance', *New Scientist*, 17 September.

32 Pang, MD, Goossens, GH, Blaak, EE (2021), 'The impact of artificial sweeteners on body weight control and glucose homeostasis', *Front Nutr*, Jan 7;7:598340.

33 Berry, S (2012), 'The sweet solution?' *The Sydney Morning Herald*, 10 December.

34 Igbinedion SO, Ansari J, Vasikaran A, Gavins FN, Jordan P, Boktor M, Alexander JS (2017), 'Non-celiac gluten sensitivity: All wheat attack is not celiac', *World J Gastroenterol*, Oct 28;23(40):7201–7210. doi: 10.3748/wjg.v23. i40.7201. PMID: 29142467; PMCID: PMC5677194.

35 Press release (2020), 'Celiac disease linked to common chemical pollutants', NYU Langone Health, https://nyulangone.org/news/ celiac-disease-linked-common-chemical-pollutants.

36 'The Oscar Mayer brand's most iconic product undergoes major quality improvements for the love of hot dogs', Business Wire, https://www.businesswire.com/news/home/20170501005499/en/ Oscar-Mayer-Brand%E2%80%99s-Iconic-Product-Undergoes-Major.

37 Ferreira, S, Sanchez, G, Alves, M, Fraqueza, M (2021), 'Natural compounds in food safety and preservation', *Sec. Nutrition and Food Science Technology*, Vol 8, https://doi.org/10.3389/fnut.2021.759594.

38 Rutzerveld, C (2014), 'Edible growth: The use of additive manufacturing technologies to create an edible ecosystem', https://www.chloerutzerveld.com/ edible-growth.

39 FSANZ (2019), 'Food colours', Food Standards Australia New Zealand, https://www.foodstandards.gov.au/consumer/additives/foodcolour.

40 Pollock, I, Warner, JO (1990), 'Effects of artificial food colours on childhood behaviours', Archives of Disease in Childhood, 65:74–77.